BMA

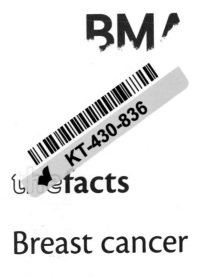

KT-430-836

the facts

Breast cancer

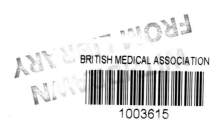

BRITISH MEDICAL ASSOCIATION

1003615

➲ also available in the**facts** series

ADHD (2nd ed.) | 9780199565030

Alcoholism (4th ed.) | 9780199231393

Alzheimer's and Other Dementias | 9780199596553

Angina and Heart Attack | 9780199599288

Ankylosing Spondylitis | 9780192632821

Asthma | 9780199211265

Autism and Asperger Syndrome | 9780198504900

Back Pain | 9780199561070

Borderline Personality Disorder | 9780199202966

Breast Cancer | 9780199558698

Chronic Fatigue Syndrome (2nd ed.) | 9780199233168

COPD | 9780199563685

Cosmetic Surgery | 9780199218820

Cystic Fibrosis (4th ed.) | 9780199295807

Depression (2nd ed.) | 9780199602933

Diabetes | 9780199232666

Down Syndrome (3rd ed.) | 9780199232772

Dyslexia and Other Learning Difficulties (3rd ed.) | 9780199691777

Eating Disorders (7th ed.) | 9780198715603

Epilepsy (3rd ed.) | 9780199233687

Epilepsy in Women | 9780199548835

Essential Tremor | 9780199211272

Facts and Practice for A-level: Biology | 9780199147663

Falls | 9780199541287

Head Injury | 9780199218226

Heart Disease | 9780199582815

Huntington's Disease (2nd ed.) | 9780199212019

Infertility | 9780199217694

Inflammatory Bowel Disease | 9780199230716

Insomnia and Other Adult Sleep Problems | 9780199560837

Living with a Long-term Illness | 9780198528821

Lung Cancer (3rd ed.) | 9780199569335

Lupus (2nd ed.) | 9780199213870

Motor Neuron Disease | 9780199206919

Multiple Sclerosis | 9780199652570

Muscular Dystrophy (3rd ed.) | 9780199542161

Myotonic Dystrophy (2nd ed.) | 9780199571970

Obsessive–Compulsive Disorder (4th ed.) | 9780199561773

Osteoarthritis | 9780199211388

Osteoporosis | 9780199215898

Panic Disorder (3rd ed.) | 9780199574698

Polycystic Ovary Syndrome | 9780199213689

Post-traumatic Stress (2nd ed.) | 9780198758112

Prenatal Tests and Ultrasound | 9780199599301

Prostate Cancer (2nd ed.) | 9780199573936

Psoriatic Arthritis | 9780199231225

Pulmonary Arterial Hypertension | 9780199582921

Schizophrenia (3rd ed.) | 9780199600915

Sexually Transmitted Infections (3rd ed.) | 9780199595655

Sleep Problems in Children and Adolescents | 9780199296149

Stroke | 9780199212729

The Pill and Other Forms of Hormonal Contraception (7th ed.) | 9780199565764

Thyroid Disease (4th ed.) | 9780199205714

Tourette Syndrome (2nd ed.) | 9780199298198

the**facts**

Breast cancer

SECOND EDITION

CHRISTOBEL M. SAUNDERS AO

Professor of Surgical Oncology, University of Western Australia, Perth, Australia

SUNIL JASSAL

Breast and General Surgeon, Melbourne Breast and Endocrine Surgeons, Australia

ELGENE LIM

Senior Medical Oncologist, Garvan Institute of Medical Research, and associate professor of Medicine, University of New South Wales, Australia

WITHDRAWN FROM LIBRARY

OXFORD
UNIVERSITY PRESS

List of abbreviations

ADH	atypical ductal hyperplasia
AI	aromatase inhibitor
ALH	atypical lobular hyperplasia
BMI	body mass index
CT	computed tomography
DCIS	ductal carcinoma in situ
DIEP	deep inferior epigastric perforator
DNA	deoxyribonucleic acid
ER	oestrogen receptor
FNA	fine needle aspiration
GnRH	gonadotrophin-releasing hormone
HER2	human epidermal growth factor
HRT	hormone replacement therapy
IDC	invasive ductal carcinoma
ILC	invasive lobular carcinoma
IVF	in vitro fertilization
LABC	locally advanced breast cancer
LCIS	lobular carcinoma in situ
LD	latissimus dorsi
LH	luteinizing hormone
LVI	lymphovascular invasion
MDM	multidisciplinary meeting
MRI	magnetic resonance imaging
NOS	not otherwise specified
NST	no specific type
OCP	oral contraceptive pill
PAP	profunda artery perforator
PARP	poly-ADP ribose polymerase
PET	positron-emission tomography
PR	progesterone receptor
SNB	sentinel lymph node biopsy

List of abbreviations

TAM	tamoxifen
TIL	tumour-infiltrating lymphocytes
TRAM	transverse rectus abdominis muscle

1

Who is at risk of breast cancer, when, and what you can do about it

⮕ Key points

- One in eight Western women will develop breast cancer
- Key risk factors include:
  - Increasing age
  - Multiple family members with breast or ovarian cancer
  - Previous atypical breast biopsy
  - Use of hormone replacement therapy (HRT)
  - Breast tissue density
  - Moderate or excess alcohol consumption
  - Obesity
  - Some ethnic groups including European (Ashkenazi) Jews
- You can reduce your risk of breast cancer
- Genetic testing identifies inherited breast cancer genes in only about 1% of people

Introduction

Breast cancer is one of the commonest cancers affecting women. Although a woman's chance of developing breast cancer (the incidence of the disease) is not increasing in most developed countries, the absolute numbers of women developing it are. This is because there are both more people in the world, and it is an ageing population—in fact around one in three people will develop some kind of cancer in their lifetime.

Another reason breast cancer may seem to be increasingly common is that it is so often in the media—whether because of a celebrity having been affected, or via campaigns to raise awareness and raise funds for research and support. Thus, when diagnosed with breast cancer, people often feel news of it is everywhere.

In most developed countries around one in eight women will develop breast cancer in their lifetime. For those who do develop it, one of their first questions is 'why me?' Predicting who is more at risk of getting breast cancer, and importantly why they are at increased risk, potentially allows an individual to alter this risk, allows health services to manage these higher risk women better, for example, through different screening programmes, and opens the way for scientists to discover how to actually prevent breast cancer.

In order to start to understand risk it is important to understand what a cancer is and how it develops.

Cancer comes about when the checks and balances, which normally make cells grow and die in an orderly fashion, get disrupted. Cells no longer accurately repair their DNA, and the body's immune system no longer mops up abnormal cells. The cause of these disruptions can be simply degeneration with age—so getting older is one of the commonest risk factors for developing breast cancer (see Fig. 1.1). Alternatively, several harmful outside influences accumulating with age, such as toxins in food and exposure to radiation (including sunlight), may be the cause. It appears some people are born with faults in their cell repair mechanisms and are more susceptible to these toxic influences. A classic example of this is an inherited fault in the *BRCA* genes, which normally control DNA repair.

Family history of breast cancer

In 2013 the actress Angelina Jolie announced she had undergone a preventative double mastectomy as she carried an inherited gene fault—a *BRCA1* mutation. She revealed her mother had died from ovarian cancer, also related to the gene fault. Angelina had been advised that she had up to an 80% chance of developing breast cancer and up to 50% chance of developing ovarian cancer, so she took pre-emptive action.

We have known about these gene faults or cancer predisposing genes (such as *BRCA1* and *BRCA2*) for more than 20 years, and it is recognized that

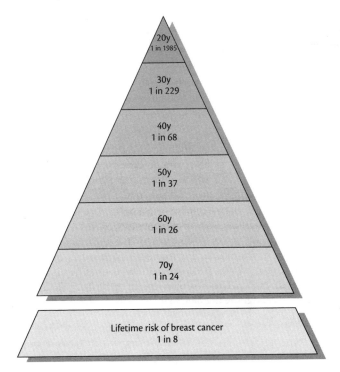

Fig. 1.1 Probability of a woman developing breast cancer within the next 10 years.

around 1% of the population carry these (higher in some ethnic groups such as Ashkenazi Jewish people). Typically, affected families will have four or five members with breast cancer who may have developed it at quite a young age (under 40 years), sometimes also ovarian cancer, and occasionally a male with breast cancer. Sometimes such family history is not evident. When there is concern, families can be referred to familial cancer services—usually part of Genetics Services, which deal with a range of inherited conditions people, including children, are born with. Counselling may be offered along with a blood test to try to determine if a breast cancer gene mutation is present.

Breast cancer risk can be reduced via a healthy weight and diet and regular exercise. Some drugs such as tamoxifen, and in older women, aromatase inhibitors such as anastrazole or exemestane may also decrease breast cancer risk. Newer drugs such as Denosumab are being trialled (see Chapter 15), which may even be useful in those with *BRCA* gene faults.

Women who have a strong family history are advised to undergo regular checks. Screening tests will usually involve a mammogram and sometimes magnetic resonance imaging (MRI) and/or ultrasound scans each year from age 30 or 5–10 years prior to the age of the youngest affected relative—whichever comes first. Regular breast self-examination can also maximize the chance a cancer will be found early.

The only sure-fire way at present to prevent cancer is to remove the breasts with a preventative mastectomy. This can be combined with immediate breast reconstruction (see Chapter 6). As the *BRCA1* and *2* gene mutations are also associated with a significant lifetime risk of ovarian cancer, it is routine to also have a discussion about removing the ovaries and fallopian tubes (which connect the ovaries to the womb) to prevent ovarian cancer.

Many more than this small percentage of the population with a detected gene fault will have some family history of breast cancer (see Fig. 1.2)—this may just be because breast cancer is so common that most families will have experienced it. But it may also be due to other inherited factors, which do not confer such a strong risk as a *BRCA* gene mutation, but nevertheless increase the risk of breast cancer. These women should seek advice from their doctor who may recommend more frequent breast checks, advice on diet, weight, and

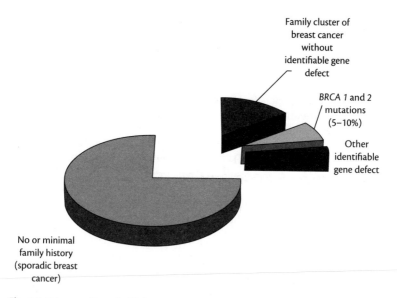

Fig. 1.2 Women affected with breast cancer.

exercise, and sometimes when the risk is moderate or high, drug treatments as mentioned here may be considered.

For women newly diagnosed with cancer it can be important to discover if this cancer is linked to a gene fault, as this may affect the treatment offered. This is more likely if a woman develops breast cancer under 40 years and if the cancer is a particular type called triple negative breast cancer. These women can be assessed by a genetic clinic and undergo a genetic blood test.

Hormone replacement therapy

Around the menopause, falling levels of female hormones made by the ovaries frequently cause unpleasant and sometimes debilitating symptoms. These can include hot flushes and night sweats, fatigue and poor concentration, a falling sex drive, and vaginal symptoms. HRT can help with some of these and is a very reasonable option for some women. However, most types of HRT (and especially those that contain progesterone) will slightly increase a woman's chance of developing future breast cancer. The risk is presumed similar whether standard HRT, 'bioavailable' or 'natural' HRT preparations are prescribed. In light of this, it is recommended that HRT is used only for significant symptoms and preferably for less than five years. Oestrogen-only HRT can be safely used for longer but poses an increased risk for uterine (womb) cancer and is thus only suitable for women with prior hysterectomy.

For women who develop breast cancer while receiving HRT, the general recommendation is to stop taking it.

Other hormone medications such as the oral contraceptive pill (OCP) can also potentially slightly increase risk, and the recommendation is usually to stop it in the context of developing a breast cancer.

What a mammogram tells us about risk: Mammographic density

Around 1 in 20 women will have very dense breasts on a mammogram—this means the X-ray looks very white—indicating more fibrous and gland tissue in the breast than fat. Younger women often have denser breasts and HRT can also increase breast density. This creates two issues for breast cancer risk and detection. Women with very high density may be up to five times more likely to get breast cancer. And secondly, breast cancers that develop in dense breasts are often hard to pick up on a mammogram; like looking for the proverbial snowball in a snowstorm! (See Fig. 1.3.)

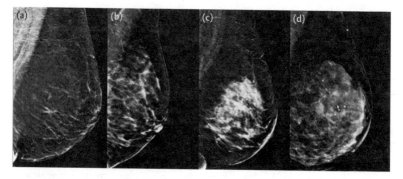

Fig. 1.3 Mammograms and breast density: (a) fatty breast; (b) some breast density; (c) more breast density; (d) dense breast.

Reprinted with permission from Wang AT, Vachon CM, Brandt KR, *et al.* Breast density and breast cancer risk: a practical review. *Mayo Clin. Proc.* 2014;89:548–57. © 2014 Mayo Foundation for Medical Education and Research. Published by Elsevier Inc. All rights reserved.

The problem is that there is currently no one accepted test for how to best measure density on mammograms and so a density score may vary between radiologists reading the mammogram. Moreover, even if a woman does have dense breasts we are not really sure which additional tests (such as perhaps an ultrasound) are best to add as a screening test. Given the uncertainty, most government-funded breast cancer screening programmes do not offer tests other than mammogram in the first instance.

If you have dense breasts on a mammogram, talk to your doctor about how you can reduce your risk of breast cancer and whether additional screening tests are warranted.

Lifestyle

As with many other diseases, breast cancer is associated with being overweight, consuming excess alcohol (two standard units or glasses per day is the max-imum recommended), and with lack of regular exercise. Of course, this does not mean that women who do not conform to this lifestyle will get cancer or indeed that a woman who does all the 'right things' will never develop cancer—rather, by living a healthy life you can reduce your chances and generally feel better as well! Although many diets are proposed as reducing breast cancer risk, in fact no specific evidence exists that one is superior to another, as long as a healthy weight and nutrition are maintained.

The recommendations are to keep your weight below a body mass index (BMI) of 25, consume less than two standard drinks of alcohol per day, and exercise strenuously for at least 30 minutes daily.

Populations where women have many children and spend much of their adult life breastfeeding also have lower risk; however, for an individual, having a few or no children and breastfeeding for little or no time does not cause breast cancer—and it is not recommended to have many children to protect against it!

Non-cancer breast conditions that increase cancer risk

Benign breast conditions such as cysts, fibroadenomas, and tender breasts with menstruation are very common and do NOT increase breast cancer risk. There are however several benign changes which can increase risk but are only found after a biopsy for something seen on a mammogram. Generally, these changes do not cause any symptoms but we know are associated with an elevated future risk of developing breast cancer. These 'lesions' include a range of changes in the cells lining the breast ducts and lobules where milk is made. The 'ductal' and 'lobular' cells have undergone changes which make them turn over too quickly and look abnormal under the microscope. They are known as proliferative changes, and in some cases are even called *in situ* cancer—where the cells themselves look cancerous, but have not yet formed a lump which can spread beyond the breast. Treatment usually consists of removing the lesion and/or yearly screening tests rather than the more usual two- or three-yearly recommendation. Some women may also be offered antihormone medication to lower their risk.

Geography

Women from different parts of the world have differing risks for breast cancer. It seems to be a disease of developed countries such as North America, Western Europe, and Australia, although it is rapidly increasing where wealth is increasing—such as in India and Eastern Europe. This is probably because a whole mixture of the aforementioned risk factors are coming into play—women are living long enough to get the disease, are starting their periods earlier, having less children, taking hormones, and getting heavier.

It is interesting to look at the risk of breast cancer in women who are born and brought up in, for example, Japan (very low risk) compared to their descendants who emigrate to the West and their descendants who are born and brought up in the West—risk progressively increases across each generation until it becomes Western.

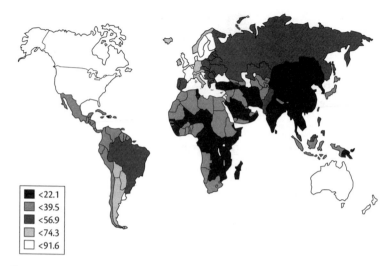

Fig. 1.4 Geography and breast cancer risk. Breast cancer incidence worldwide: age-standardized rates (world population).

Reproduced with permission from Ferlay J, Bray F, Pisani P, & Parkin DM, GLOBOCAN 2000: *Cancer Incidence, Mortality and Prevalence Worldwide. IARC Cancer Base No. 5. [1.0]* Lyon, France: IARC 2001 with permission from Wiley.

Figure 1.4 illustrates the geographical areas of the world with the highest number of newly diagnosed cases of breast cancer (shown in white) and the geographical areas with the lowest number of newly diagnosed cases (shown in dark grey).

Myths about breast cancer risk

Figure 1.5 summarizes common myths about the risk of developing breast cancer.

What you can do to protect yourself from breast cancer

Understand your risk and when this starts to climb. Institute a plan to maximize the chance of detecting any breast cancer early; early detection increases the chances for curative treatment.

For most women, this means living a healthy life, avoiding or minimizing HRT use after menopause, and undergoing regular breast imaging from 50 years of age. A two- or three-yearly screening (i.e. when you have no breast concerns)

MYTH		VERDICT
Breast cancer can be caused by an injury to the breast – a fall or a knock.	☒	Injury does NOT cause cancer but may draw the woman's attention to a lump.
Deodorants and anti-perspirants contain toxins which increase breast cancer risk.	☒	There is NO evidence that deodorants cause breast cancer.
Wearing a tight-fitting bra will cause breast cancer.	☒	Tight-fitting bras DO NOT cause breast cancer.
Women with larger breasts have a higher risk of developing cancer.	?	Risk will increase in women who are overweight but breast size alone has not been shown to be a risk factor.
Mammograms can cause breast cancer by 'squeezing' the breast or radiation exposure.	☒	Mammography is safe and effective in screening for breast cancer.
Women with silicone breast implants are not able to have a mammogram.	☒	Implants can make mammography slightly more difficult but it is still both possible and a very effective way of screening for breast cancer.

Fig. 1.5 Myths about the conditions for breast cancer risk.

mammogram from age 50 is shown to reduce the risk of dying from breast cancer. The evidence for screening mammogram prior to age 50 in the standard population is controversial. There may be some benefit in starting from 45—though if there is a protective benefit, it is likely to be small.

If you feel you may be at above average risk from breast cancer based on personal or family factors, you should discuss your situation with your local doctor and then perhaps a breast specialist. Earlier or more intensive screening tests may be warranted. For those at high risk of breast cancer, family genetic testing is sometimes performed, and preventative strategies such as drug prevention of breast cancer, prophylactic mastectomy, and even inducing early menopause via ovary removal may be options.

Preventing breast cancer

◆ Healthy diet

◆ Regular exercise

- ◆ Ideal weight
- ◆ Reduce alcohol intake
- ◆ Minimize HRT use
- ◆ Those at high risk can also consider:
  - ◆ Genetic assessment
  - ◆ Hormone depleting treatments (see Chapter 8)
  - ◆ Prophylactic breast and/or ovarian surgery

Early detection of breast cancer

- ◆ Screening mammogram two- to three-yearly from age 50
- ◆ Screening breast ultrasound and/or MRI in selected women
- ◆ Breast self-examination in higher risk women

Further resources

Breast Cancer Network Australia. *Breast Health and Awareness*. Available at: https://www.bcna.org.au/breast-health-awareness/

Breastcancer.org. *Being Overweight*. Available at: http://www.breastcancer.org/risk/factors/weight

Cancer Australia. *Familial Risk Assessment FRA-BOC*. Available at: https://canceraustralia.gov.au/clinical-best-practice/gynaecological-cancers/familial-risk-assessment-fra-boc

Cancer Council Australia. *Body Weight*. Available at: http://www.cancer.org.au/preventing-cancer/nutrition-and-physical-activity/body-weight.html

INFORMD. *Information FORum on Mammographic Density*. Available at: http://www.informd.org.au/,

Memorial Sloan Kettering Cancer Center. *Breast Cancer Screen Guidelines*. Available at: https://www.mskcc.org/cancer-care/types/breast/screening/screening-guidelines-breast

National Institute for Health and Care Excellence (NICE) (2013). *Familial Breast Cancer: Classification, Care and Managing Breast Cancer and Related Risks in People with a Family History of Breast Cancer*. Clinical guideline [CG164]. Available at: https://www.nice.org.uk/guidance/cg164

Susan G. Komen. *Breast Density on a Mammogram*. Available at: http://ww5.komen.org/Breastcancer/Highbreastdensityonmammogram.html

2

Healthy breasts

 Key points

- Be 'breast aware' (know your breasts!)

- It is normal for breasts to change throughout the menstrual cycle

- Breast tenderness is common, and alone, rarely indicates cancer

- Screening mammograms from age 50 are safe and may increase the detection of early breast cancers so potentially reduce your risk of dying of breast cancer

- Breast ultrasound is not a good screening tool

- Any persisting breast symptom or change requires medical advice—screening mammogram alone is not adequate

Breast awareness

Is there a 'normal' breast all women should have? Of course not. But many women are concerned their breasts are too lumpy, very tender, or not equal in size. A normal breast is what is normal for each individual. This naturally varies with age and the menstrual cycle. Many women experience increased tenderness and lumpiness before a period, and some women always have lumpy breasts. Variance between left and right sides is very common.

What's important are any changes a woman notes in her breasts, which seem different to the usual ebb and flow during her menstrual cycle. Anything of concern should be reported to a doctor, who can examine the breasts and decide if further tests are required.

We use the term breast awareness to mean being comfortable with one's own breasts; their typical appearance, how they feel, and the ways in which they change over the course of a menstrual cycle, and as we age (see Fig. 2.1). When women are used to their breasts they can usually detect changes outside the normal.

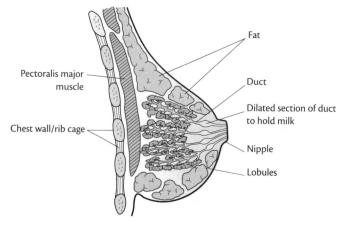

Fig. 2.1 Cross-section of a breast.

Most breast cancers are found by the woman herself, so it is important for a woman to know how to examine her own breasts (see Fig. 2.2). Many women find having this shown to them by a doctor helpful.

It is important to first LOOK. In the mirror first with the arms down then raised above the head. Look for any changes on the skin—in colour, a dimple,

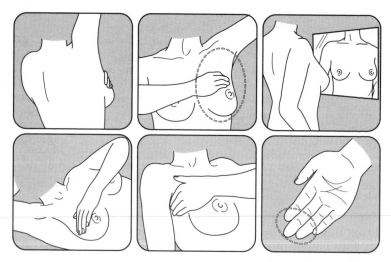

Fig. 2.2 Breast self-examination.

3

How a breast problem is investigated

> **➲ Key points**
>
> ◆ Don't panic—nine out of ten breast symptoms turn out to be from benign causes (i.e. NOT cancer)
>
> ◆ New and persisting breast symptoms or change requires a visit to the doctor, usually at least mammogram and/or ultrasound, and sometimes biopsy
>
> ◆ Breast magnetic resonance imaging (MRI) is a powerful tool in aiding breast cancer detection, but is not appropriate for all

Breast symptoms are common and nine out of ten will not be a serious condition or cancer. However, *all* persisting breast symptoms should be reported to a doctor so appropriate assessment can be performed. Assessment includes examination by a doctor, often some kind of breast imaging such as a mammogram and or ultrasound and, if a lump is found, a needle biopsy (see Fig. 3.1).

The first step will always be medical evaluation where the doctor will ask about the problem, determine if there is any particular increased risk for breast cancer in the individual, and then perform breast examination. If the doctor has any concerns at all, other tests, usually breast imaging will be organized. For most women this is a mammogram and often breast ultrasound. In very young (under 35 years) women, ultrasound alone may be ordered. But if cancer is suspected at any age, a mammogram is useful.

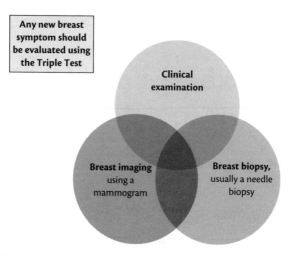

Any new breast symptom should be evaluated using the Triple Test

Clinical examination

Breast imaging using a mammogram

Breast biopsy, usually a needle biopsy

Fig. 3.1 Triple assessment of a new breast symptom.

What are the imaging tests?

Mammogram

A mammogram uses ionizing radiation (X-rays) to create a two-dimensional picture of the breast compressed between two metal plates. Typically, two views are taken—one from above and one from the side (see Fig. 3.2).

It can distinguish areas of abnormality in a breast—cancers typically appear as a white mass, often with a star-like 'spiculated' appearance (see Fig. 3.3). Clusters of tiny white calcium spots ('microcalcifications') can also indicate cancerous change. Trained doctors called radiologists read the mammogram, and can detect cancers down to half a centimetre or less in size.

Not all cancers can be seen on a mammogram, however. About 10–20% are hidden. This is especially a problem in younger women as well as some older women who have dense breast tissue where cancer can be more difficult to see. Newer technology updating the traditional mammogram is being introduced to try and improve detection of these breast cancers. Most mammogram machines will now produce digital rather than film images (much like our cameras). Three-dimensional mammography (mammogram tomosynthesis) is an exciting development which increases the chances of finding a breast cancer while decreasing the need for needle biopsy to confirm benign lesions. Other techniques including contrast ('dye') enhanced mammography and computer-aided detection are under evaluation at present.

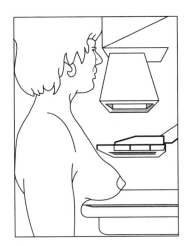

Fig. 3.2 Mammogram technique.

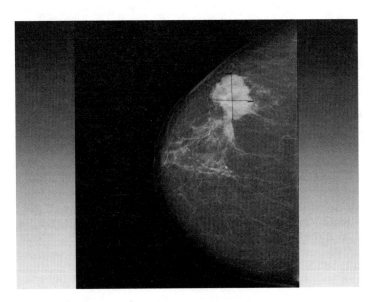

Fig. 3.3 Typical appearance of a cancer on mammogram.

Ultrasound

For many breast problems it is also recommended that a woman undergo breast ultrasound. This is a painless test using a probe on the breast which is based on detecting sound waves bouncing off different tissues in the breast tissue. It may be performed by a sonographer (a trained non-doctor technician) but is usually interpreted by a radiologist. An ultrasound is especially good at targeting a breast lump or abnormal area on mammogram. This can provide valuable additional information about the area and may determine the need for further testing—including ultrasound-guided needle biopsy (described later in this chapter). Ultrasound is also good for assessing lymph nodes under the arm, when breast cancer has been detected or is suspected. On the contrary, breast ultrasound is not a good screening tool. That is, it's not as good as mammogram for giving an overall view of the breasts.

MRI

MRI is a complex imaging test that uses strong magnetic fields to create small electrical currents which are then converted into images. This can detect differences between normal breast tissue and cancer. An injected contrast agent called gadolinium is used. Breast MRI is quite noisy and takes about 40 minutes. The woman lies on her front within a scanner with the breasts in cups underneath her. The cups are within magnetic coils, where the images are generated.

Breast MRI is a test that requires particular expertise to interpret, but in expert hands it is the most powerful imaging tool for detecting breast cancer. There are downsides though. In many countries the government does not pay for breast MRI and it can get expensive for patients. Some people who suffer claustrophobia find MRI difficult due to the length of time in an enclosed space. Importantly, along with a high detection rate for cancer, breast MRI picks up various other changes, which are not necessarily concerning, but which require further testing to definitively exclude cancer. This may lead to in retrospect 'unnecessary' anxiety, costs, and risk. We also know the contrast agent gadolinium, like all heavy metals, collects in brain tissue, although to date this has not been shown to harm human health. For these reasons, breast MRI should be used judiciously and only when mammogram and ultrasound fall short (see Fig. 3.4).

Other

Some newer types of breast imaging, such as molecular breast imaging, are showing promise. To date though, these have not been proven superior to the

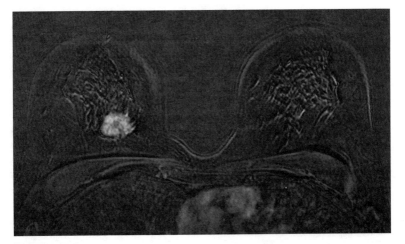

Fig. 3.4 Breast MRI.

more common breast imaging options and we are not sure of their accuracy. Other non-proven breast imaging techniques such as thermography are not recommended as the missed cancer rate may be unacceptably high.

Breast biopsies

Breast lumps or other abnormal areas such as nipple changes will usually need to have a sample taken for microscopic analysis. This is most commonly done with needle biopsy. This can be a fine needle aspiration (FNA), which collects a small sample of cells using needle and syringe, with or without local anaesthetic. The sample is sent to a pathology lab and can take up to a few days for a result. However, an FNA does not always give a definitive answer. Core biopsy is a more accurate test using a larger needle device, which actually takes a small sliver of breast tissue (a 'core') from the abnormal area. This procedure is almost always done with local anaesthetic to numb the area. Both tests are best done using mammogram or ultrasound to guide the needle (see Figs 3.5 and 3.6).

Sometimes, a larger piece of breast tissue must be removed for accurate diagnosis. This is done as a small operation under general anaesthetic by a surgeon and is called open surgical biopsy. Such a procedure is warranted when the core biopsy has provided an indeterminate result (e.g. if we're not sure needle biopsy has accurately hit the area of concern despite mammogram or

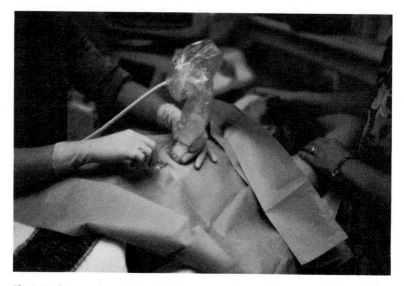

Fig. 3.5 Ultrasound-guided fine needle aspiration of the breast.

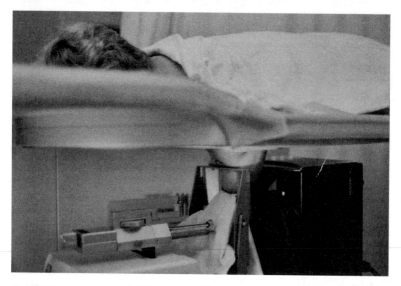

Fig. 3.6 Mammogram-guided ('stereotactic') breast core biopsy. A more technically challenging procedure than ultrasound-guided core biopsy and less comfortable for the woman. Ultrasound guidance is preferable if the lesion can be seen on both mammogram and ultrasound.

ultrasound guidance). More commonly, it may be when the lesion seen on mammogram and/or ultrasound does not seem to be cancer on needle biopsy, but we know the types of lesion seen are more commonly associated with cancer and so a larger piece of tissue is needed to exclude cancer. Lesions such as atypical hyperplasia, papillary lesions, lobular carcinoma *in situ*, and a radial scar are examples of these. We hope that with more sophisticated needle biopsy techniques being pioneered and a better understanding of these uncommon lesions, less women will require open surgical biopsy in the future to exclude cancer.

📄 Case study

Following a routine screening mammogram, Cynthia was asked to attend a breast assessment clinic as a small area of white dots or microcalcifications were seen in her left breast on the mammogram. She did not have any breast problems, nor could a lump be felt by her doctor.

The clinic repeated the mammogram on the left which confirmed a few dots of microcalcification over a centimetre area, and on the same day an ultrasound was done which was normal. It was explained by the clinic doctor that although there was a good chance this was all benign there was around a 20% chance this could be a cancer or precancerous area, so a biopsy need to be taken to confirm this.

They then went on to take a needle biopsy of the calcifications on that same day. For this Cynthia had to spend nearly an hour lying on a special table connected to the mammogram machine with her breast in a cup device. Local anaesthetic was administered and six biopsies were taken with a thin needle.

She did not need any stitches and the pain was minimal, with an ice pack, dressing, and a few paracetamol tablets needed afterwards.

Cynthia had to attend the clinic two days later for results which did indeed confirm this was a benign condition called atypical ductal hyperplasia. However, it was explained to her that even thought this is not precancerous, nor will turn into cancer, it does put her a somewhat higher risk into the future of developing a breast cancer, and a mammogram every year is recommended.

Further resources

Breastcancer.org. *Breast Cancer Tests: Screening, Diagnosis, and Monitoring*. Available at: http://www.breastcancer.org/symptoms/testing/types

Cancer Australia. *Investigating a New Breast Symptom* [Video]. Available at: https://www. youtube.com/watch?v=xZpH6yTEZBY

Cancer Australia (2006). *The Investigation of a New Breast Symptom: A Guide for General Practitioners*. Available at: https://canceraustralia.gov.au/sites/default/files/publications/ibs-investigation-of-new-breast-symptoms_50ac43dbc9a16.pdf

4

What is breast cancer?

⊃ Key points

◆ Cancer occurs when cells lose their normal 'checks and balances' and begin to grow and multiply abnormally

◆ Being a woman and increasing age are the two strongest risk factors for breast cancer

◆ *In situ* breast cancer is confined to the breast

◆ Invasive breast cancer can spread to lymph nodes and/or distant organs in the body

◆ Different breast cancers behave in different ways; it is important to understand this in determining optimum treatments for each affected woman

Introduction

Cancer (or carcinoma) is one of the common diseases that affects humans and is a major cause of both death and illness around the globe. Breast cancer is the most common cancer in women with around one in eight of us developing it in our lifetimes. It can also affect men, though much more rarely; for every 1,000 women affected by breast cancer only one man will be. Breast cancer is also more common as we age—less than 1 in 2,000 women in their twenties will develop breast cancer but from age 70, a woman has a 1 in 25 chance of cancer over the ensuing 20 years.

Ageing and femininity

These two facts immediately give us clues as to why and how breast cancer develops. Like other cancers, it is a caused by the failure of cells to properly manage the repair of the mechanisms that keep them functioning normally. While all cells of the body contain the same DNA making up our genes (except the sperm and eggs which have only half—ready to combine with each other to make a new human being), in different sites of the body the cells look different because they are only expressing the genes relevant to that site; a liver cell looks like liver but a brain cell looks like brain—even though they have all the same DNA! When controls fail, and the body's immune system fails to mop up these rogue cells, cancer can occur. Cancer's trademark is cells that can multiply and not die off naturally. They can invade adjacent tissues and eventually spread via the lymphatics to nearby lymph nodes and via the bloodstream to distant organs (see Fig. 4.1).

These failures in cell repair and control are more likely as we age because of our lifetime exposure to things in our environment which damage our DNA. Eventually, an accumulation of these damages causes mutations which are magnified in the cells, especially if these mutations occur in the area of the DNA that controls things like cell growth, division, and natural cell death. So although cancer is not inevitable as we grow older, it is more common.

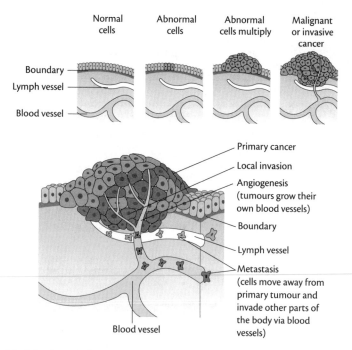

Fig. 4.1 What is cancer?

Interestingly we now know that the two commonest genes associated with familial cancer, the *BRCA1* and *2* genes, in normal cells help control DNA repair. In patients with a gene fault in *BRCA1* or *2*, where the cells are already struggling to mend themselves accurately, it takes less environmental insult to cause repair mechanisms to fail—hence cancers are more common in people with these gene faults and occur at a younger age.

The other clue to the causes of breast cancer lies in the fact that it occurs mainly in women and is associated with higher levels of female hormones—either those taken as medication such as hormone replacement therapy (HRT) or where a woman's natural hormone levels in the breast tissue may be higher, such as in obesity. It is important to understand that the tissue levels of female hormones cannot be measured with a simple blood test—the blood levels simply do not reflect both the amount of these fat-soluble hormones in tissues such as breast, nor how sensitive these tissues are to hormones.

The female hormones, oestrogen and progesterone, are important in many body processes. Cells all around the body that have receptors on them which make them sensitive to the messages these hormones are sending—messages which largely drive cells to grow and repair themselves. In the breast this is very important for the main function of breasts: to produce milk for the baby. Normal breast cells have receptors on them so they can respond to these hormones but so do most breast cancer cells. We know that quite probably all breast cancers, when they first start, will grow in response to female hormones.

Cancer in the body

We also know that cancer cells do not sit in isolation. They interact with many normal cells. These may be cells such as immune cells that recognize the cancer cells as abnormal and so are trying to destroy them. Indeed, surgically removed breast cancers with lots of immune cells within them tend to be cancers that are less likely to come back—presumably these immune cells and the wider immune system have 'learnt' what the cancer looks like and attack it when it tries to grow again.

But there are also links between cancer cells and the normal tissues of the body that seem to facilitate the growth and spread of a cancer. Cancer cells put out signals which encourage new blood vessels to grow towards them, bringing both their oxygen and food supply, and a route to spread via the blood stream. Other cells such as the supportive cells called fibroblasts seem to give out signals which can help a cancer become more mobile and spread. And platelets, the particles in blood that help us form clots, are thought to sometimes act as 'buddies' to move cancer cells around the body.

Perhaps the most bizarre of all relationships is that of the primary cancer (that is the tumour at the site it originates in—the breast for the purposes of this book) and the organs where it may spread. Essentially it would seem very hard for a cell from one organ to set up home in another—how a breast cancer can spread to and grow in the brain, for example, is something we do not understand. Yet we have some evidence that, at least in advanced disease, these host organs actually secrete substances that attract the cancer and allow it to grow in this new metastatic site.

For a breast cancer to grow and potentially spread it must have acquired a whole series of changes in its genetic makeup and indeed in other factors that modify our genes (epigenetics). Different tumours in different individuals will have their own group of changes. We are beginning to understand these 'molecular profiles' or fingerprints of tumours and are beginning to use these in clinical practice to classify cancers into subtypes. We are also beginning to understand that as a cancer spreads it does not always stay exactly the same and may acquire new gene faults or mutations, which may lead to resistance to treatments. So, for example, some tumours that are sensitive to the hormone oestrogen when a primary tumour in the breast (oestrogen-receptor (ER) positive) may become ER negative if it spreads to other sites; antihormone drugs will then not be effective against all of the cancer cells.

Understanding this complexity is not just an 'academic exercise'. We hope it will allow us to continue developing new treatments for cancer that address the specific mechanisms by which they grow and spread, and thus save patients' lives.

Classifying breast cancers

Breast cancers arise in the cells lining the milk ducts (ductal cancer) or the lobules where milk is made (lobular cancer). There are some rarer subtypes which usually reflect what the cells look like to the pathologist under the microscope. The most common subtype of breast cancer is 'ductal carcinoma NOS' (not otherwise specified).

Grade

Cancers can be graded—this reflects how aggressive the cells appear under the microscope and how unlike normal breast cells they have become. Grade 1 (low grade) tumours are the least aggressive-looking and closest in appearance to normal breast cells. Grade 2 tumours are 'intermediate' and in fact can have a range of behaviours depending on other factors. Grade 3 look the most aggressive and least like normal breast tissue. They are the faster growing tumours. *Grade is distinct from stage, which refers to how far the cancer has spread.*

Invasive and *in situ* cancer

A fundamental feature of breast cancer is that it can be what is called *in situ* or alternatively invasive cancer. Many breast cancers we find are a mixture of both. *In situ* cancers are sometimes referred to as 'precancers'. The cells look like cancer cells but are confined within milk ducts or lobules, cannot access lymphatics or blood vessels, and thus cannot spread. Invasive cancers multiply and grow through barriers in the breast—like the milk duct or lobule walls— usually forming a mass which can spread into adjacent tissues, lymphatics, and/or blood vessels, and from there to sites beyond the breast (see Fig. 4.2).

Ductal *in situ* cancer (DCIS) rarely forms a lump but most often shows up on a mammogram as tiny dots of calcium (microcalcifications) within the milk

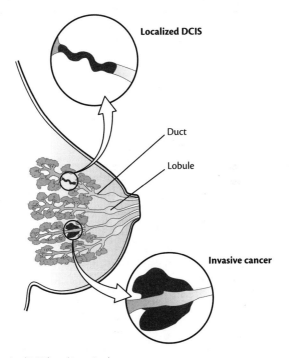

Fig. 4.2 *In situ* (DCIS) and invasive breast cancer.

ducts. Occasionally it can be in the ducts near the nipple and cause nipple discharge and bleeding. Left untreated, DCIS, especially when high grade, may go on to become invasive cancer.

Lobular carcinoma *in situ* (LCIS), in contrast, is usually a chance finding on a breast biopsy. How and when this progresses to invasive cancer is less well known, but we do know that women with this condition have up to a five times increased risk of future breast cancer in either breast and at any site in the breasts, not just where the LCIS was detected.

Lymph nodes

Lymph nodes (sometimes called lymph glands) are part of our immune system. They are all over the body, and filter and clean tissue fluid passed through them via a network of lymphatic channels (see Fig. 4.3). The fluid, now free of harmful substances such as bacteria and foreign material (e.g. tattoo dye or leaking silicon from implants), is eventually transported on and back into the blood system.

Cancer cells can spread via lymphatic channels to nearby lymph nodes. In the breast, this is most commonly nodes in the armpit, but can sometimes be

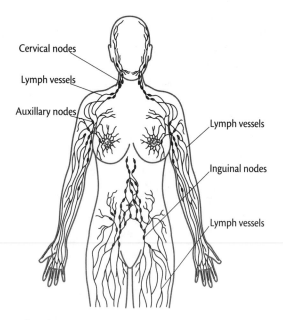

Fig. 4.3 Human lymphatic system.

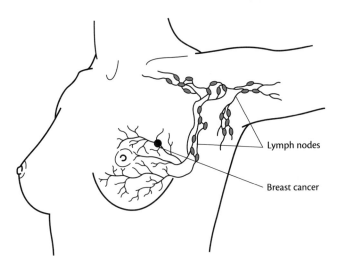

Fig. 4.4 Breast cancer and axillary lymph nodes.

nodes in the neck, chest, or abdomen (see Fig. 4.4). Most of these travelling cancer cells will be destroyed by the immune system within the lymph node, but some with specific capabilities may resist the immune defence and set up a new home, multiplying within the lymph node.

Whether or not cancer cells have spread to the lymph nodes draining a tumour is one of the most important factors in assessing how aggressively a cancer is likely to behave, and thus gives a good guide as to what treatment may be needed. If a woman has enlarged lymph nodes to feel or see on ultrasound when she is diagnosed with breast cancer, these nodes can be subjected to a needle biopsy for diagnosis. However even if lymph nodes are not apparently involved by cancer on medical examination or breast imaging, most women with invasive breast cancer will be recommended to have the nearest nodes to the breast removed to look for microscopic cancer. This is a sentinel node biopsy and is described in Chapter 6. It is part of the staging process which determines how far a breast cancer has advanced.

Tumour size

The size of a tumour may reflect how long it has been there and/or how fast it is growing. Smaller tumours are less likely to have spread than an equivalent larger tumour, and are of a better prognosis. This information, like knowledge of node involvement, helps to determine the cancer stage. A Stage 1 cancer, for

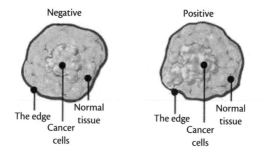

Fig. 4.5 Margins of a tumour at surgery.

example, is less than two centimetres in size and without significant spread to lymph nodes. The vast majority of these cancers are curable.

Other tumour features

Pathologists will also report on whether a tumour has spread into local blood and lymphatic vessels in the breast. This is called lymphovascular invasion (LVI) and may be an important factor in treatment recommendations beyond surgery.

Pathologists will also report on whether a tumour has been removed with a rim of normal tissue fully surrounding it—this is called the margin. Close or involved margins may mean the patient needs another operation to minimize the possibility of having left tumour in the breast (see Fig. 4.5).

Some pathology laboratories will report other tumour features such as Ki67, a marker of rapid cell turnover, or how many inflammatory and immune cells there are in a tumour. This information is harder to consider in determining what is appropriate treatment for a particular woman's cancer for two reasons. Firstly, there's no one universal way laboratories test for this information—meaning that different labs may come up with different results on the same tumour. In addition, we are still learning about the significance of this added cancer information and how it should best guide treatment decisions.

Receptors

Breast cancer cells will often be sensitive to the female hormones oestrogen and progesterone. This is measured by the amount of hormone receptors within the cell. Oestrogen-sensitive cancer cells express the hormone receptors, the ER and progesterone receptor (PR). Pathologists test for this and report the percentage of cells with these receptors and the intensity for which the receptors are seen. This is known as ER and/or PR positive cancer. We know tumours that have these receptors on the whole are less aggressive cancers and will respond to antihormone therapy (see Chapter 8).

Pathologists will also report on the degree of expression of growth receptors called HER2 (human epidermal growth factor) on the cancer cells. These can be measured by the degree of protein expression on the cell surface. Alternatively, or in addition, a more exact test is used whereby the pathologist looks for the degree of HER2 gene amplification using a test called *in situ* hybridization. About 10–15% of breast cancers overexpress HER2. Patients with this type of cancer will benefit from a group of drugs that specifically target the HER2 protein, and thus HER2 positive breast cancer cells (see Chapter 8).

Based on these receptors, breast cancers can be broadly classified into the following subtypes: (1) hormone-receptor-positive breast cancers, which comprise approximately 70% of breast cancers; (2) HER2-positive breast cancers, which comprise approximately 15–20% of all breast cancers; and (3) triple negative breast cancers (TNBC, which means that the cancer does not express ER, PR, and HER2), which comprise approximately 10% of all breast cancers.

Hormone-receptor-positive breast cancers are generally associated with relatively better outcomes. Importantly, endocrine therapies can be used for the treatment of this subtype. HER2-positive breast cancers are typically associated with a higher grade and are historically associated with relatively poorer outcomes. Anti-HER2 therapies in combination with chemotherapy have revolutionized the management of this subtype, and improved outcomes in patients significantly. Unfortunately, there are no targeted therapies that have been approved for use in patients with TNBC, which is associated with relatively poorer outcomes. Chemotherapy is therefore usually the only mode of systemic therapy. These cancers are more common in very young women and particularly in women who carry *BRCA1* inherited mutations.

Molecular profiling

Several commercial tests are now available which give a more detailed look at the genes within breast cancer cells that determine risk of cancer recurrence in patients with early-stage breast cancer. These include Oncotype, Mammaprint, Prosigna, and Endopredict. Some of these tests also help identify patients who may gain benefit from the addition of chemotherapy to their treatment. These are known as molecular profiling tests and are most likely to be useful if a tumour looks 'middle of the road' on conventional pathology testing, making it difficult to judge how aggressively or not the cancer might behave and in turn, how beneficial chemotherapy may be. Whether adding these tests to conventional pathology actually improves patient outcomes is still the subject of several very large studies worldwide. Consequently, in many countries these tests are not funded by government or health insurers and cost many thousands of dollars (or equivalent). Ordering such tests thus needs very careful consideration by the patient and her doctor as to whether it will give her additional information which could prove useful to guide treatment.

How pathology helps decide on treatment

In the following chapters, the various treatments available for breast cancer will be described in detail. All of these treatments will be guided by the pathology report of the breast cancer both from initial needle biopsy and/or after surgical removal. Size, margins, and nodal information largely guide surgical options. Patients with hormone-receptor-positive cancers will be recommended an antihormone treatment, while those with grade 3 cancers, and cancers not exhibiting hormone receptors will usually be recommended to consider chemotherapy. The presence of the HER2 receptor means the patient should be offered an anti-HER2 drug such as Herceptin.

Breast cancer prognosis by stage and type

- Treated DCIS has a near 100% five-year survival rate

- Treated Stage 1 breast cancer has a near 100% five-year survival rate

- Treated Stage 2 breast cancer has a 95% five-year survival rate

- Treated Stage 3 breast cancer has a 75% five-year survival rate

- Treated Stage 4 (that is, spread to other body organs) breast cancer has a 25% five-year survival rate

BUT

- Tumour type also has a bearing on breast cancer prognosis

- Low- to intermediate-grade ER/PR positive tumours have a more favourable prognosis than equivalent stage intermediate- to high-grade ER/PR negative tumours

- HER2 positive tumours are more prone to relapse than HER2 negative tumours, but anti-HER2 therapy is highly effective in reducing relapse rates

- '5 year survival' just means the studies have followed patients for 5 years on average but this echoes lifetime survival rates

Further resources

American Cancer Society. *Understand Your Pathology Report: Breast Cancer.* Available at: https://www.cancer.org/treatment/understanding-your-diagnosis/tests/understanding-your-pathology-report/breast-pathology/breast-cancer-pathology.html

Breast Cancer UK. *Science and Research.* Available at: http://www.breastcanceruk.org.uk/science-and-research/

Cancer Australia. *Diagnosis of Early Breast Cancer.* Available at: https://canceraustralia.gov.au/affected-cancer/cancer-types/breast-cancer/diagnosis/diagnosis-early-breast-cancer/what-does-pathology-report-mean

UCSF Health. *Basic Facts About Breast Health: Breast Cancer Biology.* Available at: https://www.ucsfhealth.org/education/breast_health/breast_cancer_biology/

5

Treating breast cancer

 Key points

- Most women with breast cancer are diagnosed early

- Treatment for early breast cancer is highly effective and usually curative

- Multidisciplinary care optimizes outcomes

- Treatment needs to focus both on the obvious cancer, and the possibility of hidden cancer deposits

- Mastectomy and/or chemotherapy is often not required

- A good breast care team treats the whole woman—not just her breast cancer!

Early breast cancer

The vast majority of breast cancer is not only treatable, but curable. More than 80% of women in developed countries are successfully treated. Most women who present with a breast symptom that turns out on testing to be breast cancer will have early stage breast cancer—that is disease confined to the breast and/or armpit lymph nodes. The next few chapters will describe available treatments for early breast cancer.

The 'journey' that a person diagnosed with breast cancer embarks on is often quite a long and complex one. There are several tests to make the diagnosis, and treatments, which may include some combination of surgery, radiotherapy, and drug therapy—often continue for many years. Then there is follow-up with regular breast imaging to make sure disease does not return and to guard against a new breast cancer.

Side effects of the cancer and its treatment, as well as the psychological impact of a cancer diagnosis, will probably have long-lasting consequences for the patient and her family.

Multidisciplinary care

In good treatment centres, a multidisciplinary team of specialists manages patients with breast cancer. It is made up from a range of health professionals which can include the breast (and sometimes plastic or reconstructive) surgeon, oncologists who deliver radiotherapy and drug treatments, doctors involved in diagnosis (pathologists and radiologists), specialist nurses, physiotherapists, and a range of others with skills in areas which may or may not be needed by an individual patient (see Fig. 5.1). In addition, a patient's general practitioner often has a critical role in the initial diagnosis and long-term aftercare but is also well positioned to aide with advice and support around treatment decisions and in acute problems associated with treatment itself. A skilled team working together and liaising closely with the patient's general practitioner means the patient has the best healthcare and optimal outcome.

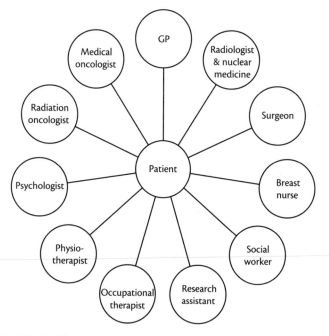

Fig. 5.1 Multidisciplinary care.

This team approach reflects how we treat breast cancer. We use a variety of treatments delivered by a range of clinicians and supported by various others with wide ranging expertise.

Breast nurses

Most breast units will have specialist breast nurses. They are highly trained in caring for people with breast cancer and can offer support, information, and care specific to the patient's needs, and often help navigate the 'journey' of breast cancer management. Breast nurses provide an easy-to-access and sometimes less confronting person to seek help from. They can help with issues from specialist bras and prostheses after surgery to the hormonal effects of treatment, and relationship and economic stresses that a cancer diagnosis may precipitate. Women often feel more comfortable discussing some issues with the breast nurse rather than their doctors.

Breast surgeon

The surgeon is usually the first specialist a patient sees at diagnosis. Breast surgeons are specialist surgeons who trained in general surgery but have extra training in managing breast disease and often reconstruction of the breast. Many countries now have registries of breast specialist surgeons and it is accepted that outcomes are usually better for the patient if they are managed by such a surgeon.

The treatment plan

At diagnosis, with the surgeon (and often in consultation with a multidisciplinary team), an initial treatment plan is made. The idea is to eradicate the obvious (or known) cancer in the body—in the breast plus or minus lymph nodes—while also mopping up any potential 'invisible' disease, which may already have spread to other parts of the body.

Treatment to the breast (local therapy) and lymph nodes (regional therapy) is primarily with surgery and often radiotherapy. Treatment for the whole body (systemic therapy) involves drug treatments, both oral and intravenous. By treating both the known cancer (with local and regional therapy), but also the potential of hidden, microscopic cancer (with systemic therapy), we can significantly reduce the chance of a breast cancer ever returning.

For most women with early breast cancer, surgery is the first treatment offered. This both removes the known breast cancer in a woman's body and also gathers more information about the cancer—via the pathologist's assessment of the tumour in the laboratory. This extra information can be very helpful in determining what further treatments may be worthwhile in reducing the risk of cancer recurrence.

Some women may be offered drug treatment before surgery. This is called neoadjuvant treatment and is usually chemotherapy, but occasionally endocrine therapy (also known as hormonal therapy). The advantage of this approach is most pronounced in women with larger tumours, and women with triple negative and HER2-positive subtypes of breast cancer. In these patients, it is highly likely they will be recommended chemotherapy anyway after surgery. Giving it before may shrink the tumour or even make it completely disappear. This allows for a smaller and potentially more effective operation. It also means that both patient and doctor can actually measure if the drugs are working on the cancer by watching the tumour for shrinkage. This will be discussed in detail in Chapter 8.

Most patients with early breast cancers will have no visible or measurable disease elsewhere, and so imaging the whole body for cancer is not helpful. However, breast cancer can spread to other parts of the body. In some women with more aggressive early breast cancer it is important to exclude this by doing tests which look at the commonest sites of spread—including lungs and liver (with a computed tomography (CT) scan) and bones (with a bone scan).

Research trials

All of our modern treatments for breast cancer have been developed as a result of research, and so many patients will be offered the option of participating in research studies of new treatments or tests we are currently developing. This can be at any stage of treatment—from new diagnostic tests, to innovative techniques in surgery, radiotherapy, supportive care, or other services and of course, new drug treatments. A committee with expertise in the ethics and conduct of research (an ethics committee or institutional review board) should always have assessed these trials.

It is very important to understand that although there may be an individual benefit in participating, it is NOT compulsory and deciding not to participate in no way changes your usual treatment or how the clinicians care for you. Many patients are, however, willing to contribute to research studies which will lead to future advances in cancer care. It is not unusual that treatment units who undertake research are often those with the most up-to-date care.

Holistic care

Another important aspect of treating breast cancer is that of treating the whole person—not just her breasts! The shock of diagnosis and concerns

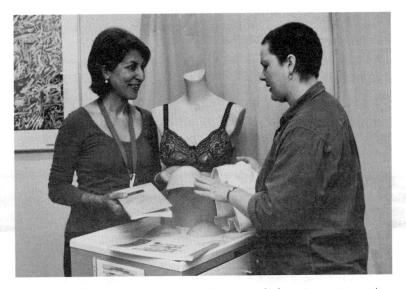

Fig. 5.2 Specialist breast nurses are an invaluable source of information, support, and comfort.

about survival, feelings of anger, isolation, and depression, the loss of libido and sexual feelings, the physical and metal consequences of treatment, as well as practical issues including change in employment and financial stress, are often interconnected and it can be artificial to try to separate them. Many of these issues will be discussed in Chapters 10 and 11, but a person reading this book has already taken a first step in improving their ability to cope with breast cancer—getting information and understanding the disease will help! (See Fig. 5.2.)

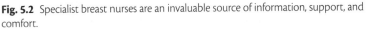 Case study

Kathy is a 46-year-old woman who has noticed a lump in her right breast for 2 months and had undergone a mammogram and ultrasound ordered by her GP, which suggested it was a breast cancer. She was referred to a specialist breast unit at her local hospital. A needle test confirmed this was a 4 cm breast cancer with at least one lymph node involved with tumour but with no obvious cancer elsewhere in the body on examining her and doing other tests including a CT and bone scan. The needle (core) biopsy had shown it to be a 'triple negative' breast cancer, which is one without receptors for female hormones or HER2.

The surgeon explained this to Kathy, and that her case was being discussed by the multidisciplinary team in their weekly patient meeting. It was suggested that Kathy be referred to a medical oncologist to find out more about having her chemotherapy before surgery, known as neoadjuvant chemotherapy. The breast nurse was present in the consultation with the surgeon but then spent some time afterwards with Kathy and her husband discussing treatment options and giving her information in both a written form and how to access useful sites on the internet. Kathy has made plans to meet again with the breast nurse the following week to go over all the information and to see what other support she may need over the coming months to help her cope with treatment and side effects.

Further resources

America Cancer Society. *Treating Breast Cancer*. Available at: https://www.cancer.org/cancer/breast-cancer/treatment.html

Cancer Council Victoria. *Treatment for Breast Cancer*. Available at: http://www.cancervic.org.au/cancer-information/cancer-types/cancer_types/breast_cancer/treatment_for_breast_cancer.html

Cancer Research UK. Treatment. Available at: http://www.cancerresearchuk.org/about-cancer/breast-cancer/treatment

6

Surgical treatments

 Key points

- Surgery is usually the first step in treatment and involves surgery to the breast, and in cases of invasive breast cancer, lymph nodes in the armpit as well

- The majority of women can, and opt to, preserve their breast and just remove the cancerous area

- If mastectomy is required, breast reconstruction can be performed at the same time or later on

- Breast-conserving surgery, when appropriate, is equivalent to mastectomy in terms of cure rates

- Cosmetic outcomes are generally very good

Breast surgery

Surgery is the first step in the treatment pathway for most women with breast cancer. The aim of surgery is to remove all the affected area of the breast and either remove lymph nodes if there is known spread of cancer to them, or sample a few to exclude this.

Breast surgery can be either removing the entire breast—a mastectomy—or just the affected area. The latter is called breast-conserving surgery, wide local excision, or in plain terms, lumpectomy. For most women having breast-conserving surgery, a course of radiotherapy to the rest of the breast will be recommended afterwards, so in fact the whole breast is treated. We know from decades of research that the outcomes in terms of both preventing cancer recurrence in the breast and indeed cure are very similar for both approaches.

So why do why do some patients have mastectomy and others breast conservation? One of the most important determinants is the patient herself. Some women are more comfortable with a complete mastectomy even if the surgeon suggests breast conservation is possible.

Breast-conserving surgery

Around 60% of women will opt for breast-conserving surgery. This means removing the cancerous area, which can be felt or seen on breast imaging, along with a surrounding rim (or 'margin') of normal breast tissue. Breast conservation is best suited to smaller lumps—broadly speaking less than 4 cm in size. But this does depend on the size of the cancer compared to the breast size and the position of the cancer within the breast. The surgeon will assess whether wide local excision can be performed while still maintaining a good breast size and shape. If not, mastectomy may be required, or sometimes it is possible to shrink a larger tumour with chemotherapy to enable successful breast conservation.

Up to a third of women with breast cancer will have it detected by mammographic screening. Most of these tumours will be small and often not able to be felt (impalpable). If a woman has undergone preoperative (neoadjuvant) chemotherapy, the tumour may have shrunk away completely. Ductal carcinoma *in situ* (DCIS) doesn't usually cause a mass at all, but still needs to be removed. To find these impalpable cancers within the breast at operation, it is necessary to mark them in some way before the operation to give the surgeon a guide to follow to know where the cancer is. There are several techniques for doing this, all of which use mammogram or ultrasound guidance. These include placing a thin wire called a hook wire into the cancer, placing a slightly radioactive marker (an iodine seed) or sometimes a carbon track to the tumour. Mostly this is done on the morning of surgery, under a local anaesthetic in the X-ray department. The surgeon can then follow the wire, radioactive trail, or carbon track to the cancerous area, which is then removed and subjected to X-ray (or ultrasound) to confirm tumour excision.

In general, breast conservation gives a woman better quality of life outcomes after surgery compared with mastectomy. There are downsides to breast conservation, however. Preoperative scans may underestimate the amount of cancer present and so the first surgery does not remove it all—that is, there are involved margins. This occurs in around one in five surgeries and usually means the patient requires further surgery, either re-excision or mastectomy.

Oncoplastic breast surgery

The aim of breast-conserving surgery is to remove the entire cancer and give the best possible cosmetic outcome. To improve this, breast surgeons have been developing what are known as oncoplastic techniques. These essentially remodel the breast tissue after the cancer has been removed (but in the same operation), giving the breast back a more natural shape with the least possible (and hopefully no) deformity. These techniques also mean quite large tumours can sometimes be removed by reducing the breast size at the same time—a bonus for many women, though it does mean that often the other breast requires surgery either at the same time or later, to achieve good symmetry.

Mastectomy

Mastectomy means removing all the breast tissue. It is often recommended for patients who have relatively large cancers, cancers involving the skin over the breast or muscles below it, or if there is extensive DCIS, which although cannot be felt, is involving many of the breast ducts which if left can become an invasive cancer. Mastectomy is also done for prevention reasons in women without breast cancer but with a very strong chance of developing it due to, for example, a family gene fault (such as a *BRCA* gene). Women may also choose mastectomy if they wish to avoid radiotherapy, or if they are particularly concerned about needing ongoing follow-up mammograms.

In fact, it is quite common for women at diagnosis to initially request a mastectomy—or even double mastectomy—in the belief that this is the best way to ensure they are cured and cancer does not come back. For most women, however, if breast conservation is possible this gives a very similar cure rate to mastectomy, and certainly removing the other (normal) breast does not increase the chance of cure at all.

Mastectomy or double mastectomy DOES reduce the chance of a second (new) cancer developing—but for most women, this risk is not overly high, perhaps around 10–15% across the lifetime. (Remember, even for women without a history of breast cancer, lifetime risk of breast cancer is around 12%.) In addition, women who've had breast cancer will be watched closely with yearly breast imaging. Any new breast cancer is likely to be picked up at an early and curable phase.

There are several different types of mastectomy—all remove the breast tissue—but it is possible to save most or all of the skin if immediate breast reconstruction is planned. Sometimes it is even reasonable to save the nipple and areola to facilitate an even more natural-looking breast reconstruction (see Fig. 6.1).

(a)

(b)

(c)

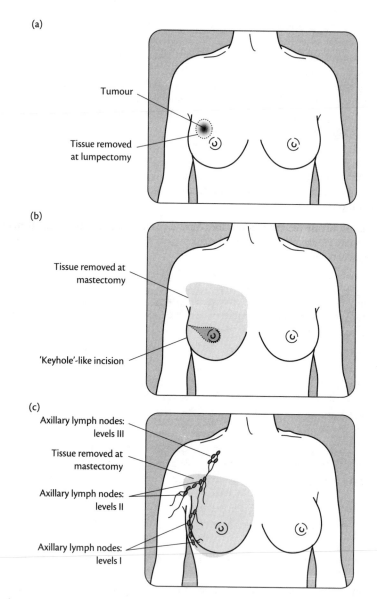

Fig. 6.1 Tissue removed during breast surgery for cancer: (a) a woman with lumpectomy; (b) A woman with skin-sparing mastectomy; (c) a woman with total mastectomy and axillary clearance.

Breast reconstruction

There are various ways of reconstructing a breast and it can be done at the time of mastectomy or at any stage down the track as a delayed reconstruction. There are several benefits to immediate reconstruction, including that of the woman not having to live without a breast. This can have significant positive psychological ramifications and in particular, may help a woman better cope with her cancer diagnosis. It is more feasible to preserve skin (and potentially nipple) if the reconstruction is done at the same time as the mastectomy, leading to a better cosmetic result. Although reconstructive surgery often requires more than one operation to achieve the ideal result, having it at the same time as a mastectomy can avoid the need for one more operation.

Delayed breast reconstruction does have a place though. Some women may not want to take on the added surgical complexity and potential delay to their cancer drug treatment that an immediate breast reconstruction sometimes entails. Sometimes there are specific treatment aspects which may also caution against immediate reconstruction. Many surgeons are reluctant to offer it if radiotherapy is expected to the chest after surgery. Radiotherapy can affect the reconstruction results by leading to a hardened implant (capsular contracture) if an implant is used, or distortion of the fat (fat necrosis) if the reconstruction is created from the body's own tissues, for example, with a deep inferior epigastric perforator (DIEP) flap. As reconstruction is often performed by a plastic surgeon, it can be difficult to schedule both a breast surgeon and plastic surgeon in the time frame needed to operate on the cancer. However, women can often experience long delays waiting for reconstruction as a second procedure as it is not classified as urgent.

Types of breast reconstruction

Breast reconstruction can use an implant placed under tissues on the chest wall, can be made entirely from the body's own skin, fat, and sometimes muscle (called a tissue flap), or can utilize a combination of both techniques. Which type of reconstruction is most suitable for an individual depends on both their body and breast shape and size, on the results required, how healthy a person is otherwise, what other treatment the patient is likely to need (such as radiotherapy) or has had, and on what the patient prefers.

Each decision will need to be tailored to the patient after discussion with the surgeons, and more detailed information can be found in 'Further resources'.

Implant based reconstruction

Implant reconstructions are usually done in two stages. Initially a temporary implant called a tissue expander is placed under the skin and muscle of the chest. It is gradually inflated either by saline through a device under

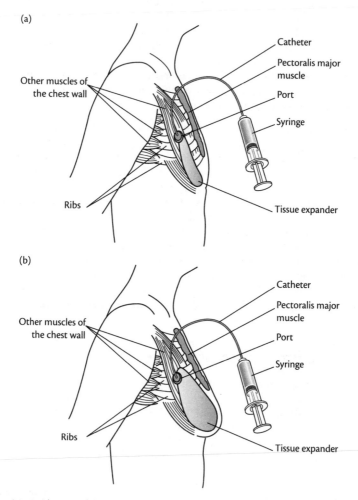

Fig. 6.2 A side view of the breast area with (a) an unfilled tissue expander in place; (b) a filled tissue expander in place.

the skin over some weeks, or may be the type which self-inflates over a similar period. This creates a pocket and at the second operation a silicone implant, which has a more natural shape and feel, is swapped into this pocket (see Figs 6.2 and 6.3). At this time a nipple and areola reconstruction can be performed.

Increasingly surgeons are using various types of synthetic or natural materials to cover the implant inside the skin. This can sometimes do away with the need for the tissue expander, whereby the final silicone implant is used at initial operation.

Implant reconstructions are the quickest and easiest option but are not ideal for all women and have significant complication rates, including the need to revise the surgery in up to a third of women.

Latissimus dorsi flap reconstruction (LD Flap)

The LD flap usually also utilizes an implant but brings the large flat back muscle called the latissimus dorsi to cover the implant. This has the advantage of allowing a larger reconstruction and often a better shape, but some women are not keen on muscle disruption—although it is usually only a very minor functional issue, with no loss of movement or power. The operation can be done by removing some back skin (thus a scar on the back) or via the mastectomy scar (Figs 6.4 and 6.5). An LD flap is a very robust reconstruction that rarely needs revision and can be done as both an immediate or delayed procedure.

Transrectus abdominis muscle (TRAM) and deep inferior epigastric perforator (DIEP) flap reconstructions

The names of these operations stand for the muscle (transverse rectus abdominus) or blood supply (deep inferior epigastric pedicle) on which they are based—the six pack, in fact!

These much larger operations use the fat of the tummy plus or minus some muscle to make a new breast, which means no implants are needed and the re-construction is made entirely from the woman's body tissues, thus will change

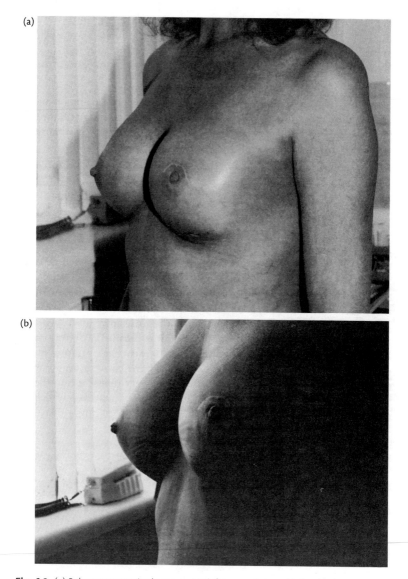

Fig. 6.3 (a) Subcutaneous nipple preserving left mastectomy with implant reconstruction and augmentation of the normal right breast. (b) Close-up of nipple preserving mastectomy and implant reconstruction.

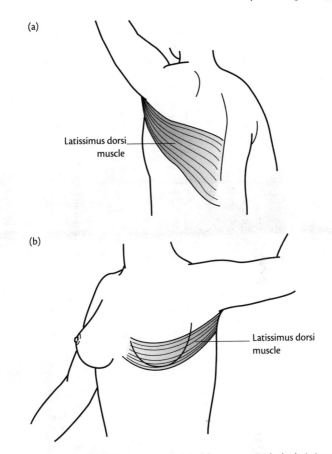

Fig. 6.4 Latissimus dorsi (LD) flap reconstruction: (a) a woman with the latissimus dorsi muscle in place; (b) a woman with the latissimus dorsi muscle swung forward to re-create the new breast.

size as she does (Fig. 6.6). It does mean a long scar on the lower tummy and is a complex procedure usually requiring microsurgery and a long hospital stay (at least a week) and recovery of at least 6 weeks. However, for fit and healthy suitable women it can give an excellent cosmetic result which is long-lasting (Fig. 6.7).

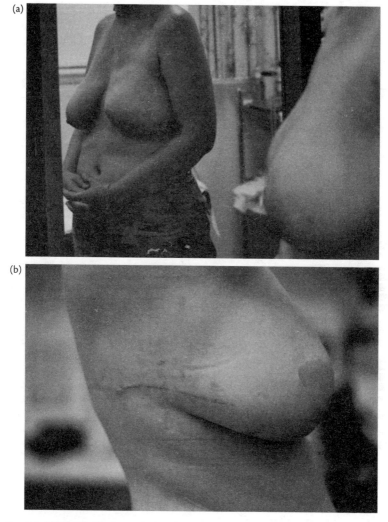

Fig. 6.5 (a) LD flap; (b) close-up of LD flap.

Other less common reconstructive options use other muscles and areas of fat to reconstruct the breast, such as the fat under the lower crease of the buttocks.

Following the reconstruction of the breast, a nipple can be made with the skin over it, which is often tattooed to achieve a realistic colour.

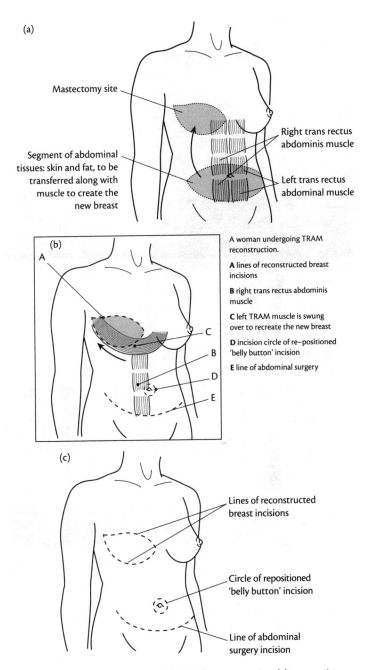

(a)

Mastectomy site

Right trans rectus abdominis muscle

Segment of abdominal tissues: skin and fat, to be transferred along with muscle to create the new breast

Left trans rectus abdominal muscle

(b)

A

C

B

D

E

A woman undergoing TRAM reconstruction.

A lines of reconstructed breast incisions

B right trans rectus abdominis muscle

C left TRAM muscle is swung over to recreate the new breast

D incision circle of re–positioned 'belly button' incision

E line of abdominal surgery

(c)

Lines of reconstructed breast incisions

Circle of repositioned 'belly button' incision

Line of abdominal surgery incision

Fig. 6.6 Transrectus abdominis muscle (TRAM) reconstruction: (a) preparation; (b) process; (c) lines of incision.

(a)

(b)

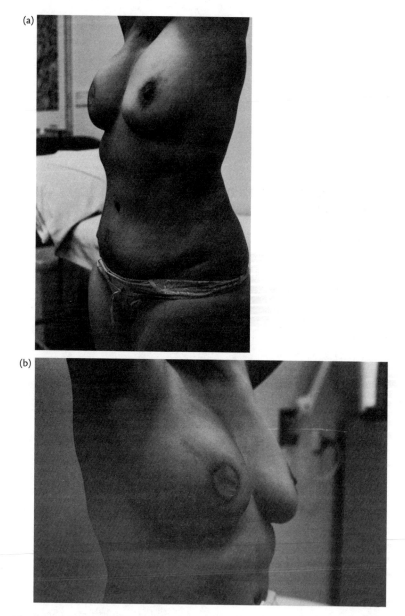

Fig. 6.7 (a) TRAM flap; (b) close-up of the TRAM flap.

The alternative to reconstruction is obviously not to have one—a very reasonable option for many women who do not wish to or cannot have extensive surgery and have the option of a prosthesis to wear in the bra.

Surgery to the opposite breast

When operating on one breast for cancer reasons, it is sometimes useful to perform surgery on the other side too in order to create a matched look. This is known as equalization surgery. It may involve a breast reduction, breast lift, or even augmentation (enlargement) surgery.

Surgery to the lymph nodes in the axilla

At cancer diagnosis, it is important to establish if the breast tumour has spread to the lymph nodes. This happens in about a quarter of women with newly diagnosed breast cancer and is one of the most important prognostic factors or indicators of how aggressive a cancer may prove to be, and thus often guides the need for treatment such as chemotherapy.

Enlarged lymph nodes containing cancer can sometimes but felt or seen on ultrasound scan, and will then be subjected to needle biopsy. If the nodes do contain cancer it is important to treat these. This is usually with surgery called an axillary clearance, although can also be with radiotherapy.

An axillary clearance is performed at the same time as the breast operation either through the same incision (cut) or a separate one under the arm. Usually some but not all nodes are removed and sent for pathology analysis. Axillary surgery can lead to both short-term complications of upper arm pain or numbness and reduced arm movement, and longer-term complications of arm swelling (lymphedema) and shoulder stiffness. It is important for a physiotherapist to give advice and treatment for this, and preventative measures can reduce complications.

If no obvious cancer has spread to the lymph nodes, most patients undergoing surgery for invasive cancer (and those undergoing mastectomy for either invasive or *in situ* cancer) will be offered a sentinel node biopsy. This procedure involves injecting one or more types of dye the day of surgery or just before, so the surgeon at operation can find the very lowest lymph node under the arm and with a small incision (or if a mastectomy is being done through the same incision) remove this one or a few nodes for pathology assessment. Conventionally, if the sentinel node contains any cancer cells the patient is offered more treatment under the arm; surgery to remove more nodes or radiotherapy.

However, it may be that the other treatments such as chemotherapy will be enough to deal with tiny amounts of residual cancer. This is indeed how chemotherapy works—it deals with tiny amounts of cancer elsewhere in the body. Studies are underway to confirm if this is the case and these patients with only small amounts of disease in the sentinel lymph nodes can avoid further surgery with its potential complications.

Removal of ovaries

Occasionally, surgical removal of the ovaries and fallopian tubes (salpingo-oophorectomy) may make up part of the hormonal treatment of breast cancer in premenopausal patients. There is also a benefit in reducing the risk of both breast and ovarian cancer in a small group of women who have a genetic risk (*BRCA 1* or *2* mutation). Oophorectomy can be done either via traditional open abdominal surgery or by 'keyhole' (laparoscopic) surgery, which means smaller cuts and a quicker recovery. Oophorectomy will cause menopause in premenopausal women and any benefits must be weighed up against this. This is discussed further in Chapter 8.

📄 Case study

Annie is a 48-year-old mother of four who noted a lump in the upper inner part of her left breast a few weeks ago. She has been found on mammogram, ultrasound, and needle biopsy to have a 2 cm cancer but with a much larger area of DCIS, and because of the position and size of the cancer has been advised that breast-conserving surgery (lumpectomy) would leave an unacceptable scar and loss of tissue. She is therefore going to have a mastectomy and wants to have a reconstruction at the same time.

She is fit and well otherwise but is a bit overweight with E cup breast, which she has always wanted to have reduced. The breast surgeon suggests she see the plastic surgeon as well to see if she is suitable for a DIEP flap reconstruction which would use her own abdominal wall fat. Although a big operation, she and her surgeons feel this would give her the best cosmetic result for her body shape and at a later operation she can have her normal right breast reduced a little to match.

After to some tests to see if the tiny blood vessels going to her abdominal fat are good enough to use for the surgery, she undergoes a skin-sparing mastectomy (and sentinel node biopsy) with a cut just around the nipple (removing it and the areola but keeping all the breast skin) and an immediate DIEP flap reconstruction. She is in hospital with drains and pain relief for

8 days (the first night in the intensive care unit for close monitoring) but recovers well and by 6 weeks is back to doing most household chores.

Ten months later, after she finishes chemotherapy, she comes back to hospital for just one night to have the other breast reduced and a nipple reconstruction to cover the scar on the left.

Further resources

Breastcancer.org. *Surgery*. Available at: http://www.breastcancer.org/treatment/surgery

Breconda. *Breast Reconstruction Decision Aid*. Available at: https://breconda.bcna.org.au

Cancer Australia. *Breast Reconstruction*. Available at: https://canceraustralia.gov.au/affected-cancer/cancer-types/breast-cancer/treatment/breast-reconstruction

Cancer Australia. *Surgery*. Available at: https://canceraustralia.gov.au/affected-cancer/cancer-types/breast-cancer/treatment/what-does-treatment-breast-cancer-involve/breast-cancer-surgery

NHS Choices. *Breast Cancer in Women: Treatment*. Available at: http://www.nhs.uk/livewell/breastcancer/pages/reconstruction.aspxNIH

NIH National Cancer Institute. *Sentinel Lymph Node Biopsy*. Available at: https://www.cancer.gov/about-cancer/diagnosis-staging/staging/sentinel-node-biopsy-fact-sheet

7

Radiotherapy

 Key points

◆ Radiotherapy reduces the risk of breast cancer returning in the treated breast quite substantially

◆ Lumpectomy plus breast radiotherapy is equivalent to mastectomy in terms of curing breast cancer

◆ Radiotherapy is almost always recommended after breast-conserving surgery for invasive breast cancer

◆ Radiotherapy is often recommended after breast-conserving surgery for ductal carcinoma *in situ* (DCIS)

◆ Side effects involve mainly the breast and can be long term

◆ Radiotherapy is sometimes recommended after mastectomy too

◆ Newer, more 'patient friendly' treatments are in the pipeline

What is radiotherapy?

Radiotherapy, or radiation therapy, is a cancer treatment which uses a type of X-ray. It involves computed tomography (CT)-guided high energy radiation delivering radioactive particles accurately to the target. In breast cancer treatment, radiotherapy is most commonly used alongside surgery in treating the breast, and sometimes nearby lymph nodes.

Radiotherapy works by destroying rapidly growing cells—like cancer cells—while having less effect on slower growing normal breast cells, which can then recover. For most people it is a well-tolerated painless treatment which involves lying flat on a bench for up to 20 minutes a day with the arm raised, while the few minutes of radiation treatment is delivered. Because the equipment to give radiotherapy is so specialized, treatment is centralized to fewer centres than other breast cancer treatments are available in.

Who gets radiotherapy?

Radiotherapy is usually given after surgery. For women who have undergone breast-conserving surgery for invasive disease, it is almost always recommended. Radiotherapy is often also recommended after lumpectomy for DCIS. This is because even though all of the known cancer has been removed, undetectable microscopic amounts may still be in the conserved breast and radiotherapy aims to destroy these. In fact, we know post-surgery radiotherapy will reduce the chance of cancer returning in the breast from around one in five to less than 2%.

Apart from to the breast after breast conserving surgery, radiotherapy to the chest wall may be recommended for some women after mastectomy. It may also be used to the armpit after removal of cancerous nodes and/or to lymph nodes higher up towards and into the neck. Simply put, radiotherapy offers a benefit in these situations if it is assessed that there is a significant risk of cancer regrowing from residual hidden microscopic cancer deposits. Women most at risk of this are those with cancer growing into breast skin or chest muscles at the outset, and those with cancerous lymph nodes. The more lymph nodes are involved, the higher the risk of cancer returning in the breast and regional lymph node area, and thus the higher the chance radiotherapy may help.

Finally, radiotherapy is also useful in women with problematic deposits of metastatic cancer—that is, cancer distant to the breast and its draining lymph nodes. While it can't be used everywhere there might be cancer as the doses required would be too toxic for the whole body, if there is a cancer spot here or there causing an acute problem, radiotherapy can bring the area under control quite rapidly. Classic areas for this type of treatment are the brain and bone.

Planning radiotherapy

The first stage of radiotherapy, after meeting the team who will deliver it, and discussing the treatment and side effects, is the planning session. This uses a simulation machine which mimics where the radiation will be delivered to. CT scanning is incorporated to help target the area very accurately. A small tattoo dot on either side of this area has traditionally been placed to create fixed points which facilitate the accurate repetitive targeting to the area required over the course of treatment. More recently, units are beginning to move away from the need for tattooing, relying instead on image-guided radiotherapy.

Treatment takes anywhere from 3 to 6 weeks, depending on the schedule decided on. Recent research has confirmed that for some women, a 3-week course is sufficient. This is called hypofractionated radiotherapy and can be

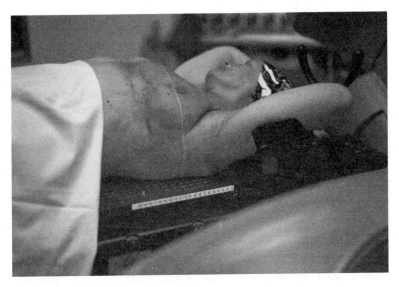

Fig. 7.1 Woman undergoing radiotherapy.

discussed with the doctor. For many women though, treatment will be daily (usually Monday to Friday) over 5 or 6 weeks. Some women receive a 'boost'— extra radiotherapy to the surgical site over a week, targeted within the breast where the highest concentration of residual cancer cells may be.

Treatment usually starts 3 weeks to 3 months after surgery, and only once the wounds are healed. If a patient is having chemotherapy, radiation treatment is delayed until after this is completed as the combination can cause unwanted side effects (see Fig. 7.1).

Common complications—skin and breast tissue

During radiotherapy the skin can feel tight and tender, and a marked 'sunburn' reaction can occur, even with blistering and skin peeling. This usually recovers within weeks, but long term the breast can remain firmer and swollen and the skin colour can be permanently changed. If the beast remains very swollen this is termed breast lymphedema and physiotherapy is very helpful. Occasionally a low-grade infection or cellulitis develops.

Local side effects are worse in women with larger breasts and those with diabetes. Radiation therapists and nurses will give advice about skin care to minimize side effects and usually recommend a moisturizer or other skin care. It is important to avoid sun exposure during treatment.

Less common complications

Radiotherapy does cause stiffness of surrounding muscles and other tissues. Although this can be treated by a physiotherapist and with good skin care, it makes delayed implant-based reconstructions more difficult as they rely on healthy pliant chest wall muscles and overlying skin.

Radiotherapy to the lymph nodes, especially if a number have been removed already, has a significant risk of arm lymphedema. Again, prevention and treatment via a lymphedema practitioner is important.

Women often complain of fatigue and sometimes depression during radiotherapy—this is not uncommon in all cancer treatments. Managing fatigue is difficult but regular exercise has been shown to help.

Longer-term serious side effects of breast radiotherapy, such as an effect on the heart and lungs and radiation-induced cancers, are uncommon but will be discussed by the specialist radiation oncologist.

Newer techniques

Breath-holding technique for left-sided breast cancers

To decrease the amount of radiation which reaches the heart, some radiotherapy machines are fitted with equipment which means the beam only activates when the lungs are filled with air, so the heart is further away from the radiation.

Intensity-modulated radiotherapy

This technique uses computers to focus the radiation beam onto a very specific area. Research is underway to see if this is more effective in breast cancer, as has been shown in other cancers.

Partial breast radiotherapy

Of the few breast cancers that do recur in the breast, most do so near the site of the first cancer—it seems logical to target the radiotherapy to this site and not irradiate the whole normal breast (indeed, we do not radiate the other breast for a cancer on one side!)

Several techniques have evolved to do this, one of the most promising of which is intraoperative radiotherapy. It has been shown to be just as effective as whole breast radiotherapy for older women with small, good outlook tumours. Instead of over many weeks, treatment is given just once, in the operating theatre at the same time as the tumour removal. At present, very few centres worldwide offer this.

Advanced and recurrent breast cancer

Radiotherapy can usually only be given once at a given site, so if a cancer returns in the breast after breast-conserving surgery and radiotherapy, mastectomy is recommended.

As mentioned already, radiotherapy is sometimes given if breast cancer is found in other parts of the body such as the bones or brain. This is discussed more in Chapter 12.

 Case study

Sunita is a 76-year-old lady who was found on a routine check by her GP to have a thickened area in the lower part of her right breast. A mammogram and needle biopsy showed this to be a small 15 mm slow-growing cancer with no apparent lymph nodes involved on an ultrasound under the arm.

Sunita has high blood pressure and diabetes but was thought fit for surgery and she was keen to keep her breast if she could.

After discussion in the multidisciplinary meeting her surgeon discussed with her the option of having the breast lump removed along with the lowest node under the arm (a sentinel node biopsy). As the hospital she was attending had the necessary equipment, she was offered intraoperative radiotherapy to the area at the same time, while under the same anaesthetic. It was explained this would take about 45 minutes extra of operating time and she may have a slightly red breast afterwards, but she hopefully would not need further radiotherapy, as long as there were no unexpected results from the pathology report. She would be recommended to have some hormone therapy (see Chapter 10). It was explained that the chance of breast cancer coming back in the breast after these procedures was very low—perhaps 2% at 5 years—although perhaps about 1% higher than with a 6-week course of radiotherapy.

She was very keen on the idea of having all local treatment at one visit, and thought the 2–3% chance of cancer returning was very acceptable as long as her quality of life remained good.

Treatment went according to plan and 6 years later Sunita remains cancer free, although as an 82-year-old now has other significant health issues but is coping well still at home with family help.

Further resources

Cancer Australia. *Radiotherapy*. Available at: https://canceraustralia.gov.au/affected-cancer/cancer-types/breast-cancer/treatment/what-does-treatment-breast-cancer-involve/radiotherapy-breast-cancer/radiotherapy-early-breast-cancer/side-effects-radiotherapy-early-breast-cancer

Cancer Research UK. *Radiotherapy for Breast Cancer*. Available at: http://www.cancerresearchuk.org/about-cancer/breast-cancer/treatment/radiotherapy

Sharecare. *What is Partial Breast Irradiation?* Available at: https://www.sharecare.com/health/breast-cancer-treatment/what-is-partial-breast-irradiation?logref=Helpful_Button&regref=Helpful_Button

8

Drug (systemic) therapy for early breast cancer

 Key points

- Systemic treatments are given to minimize the chance of cancer returning either in the breast or elsewhere in the body

- Systemic therapy can be given before surgery (neoadjuvant therapy) or after surgery (adjuvant therapy)

- Endocrine therapies are recommended for all patients with oestrogen-receptor (ER) and/or progesterone-receptor (PR) positive tumours

- Bisphosphonates may benefit post-menopausal women with ER- and/or PR-positive tumours

- HER2-targeted therapies are recommended for patients with HER2-positive tumours

- Chemotherapy is a large group of different drugs which target faster-growing cancer cells. It is usually given over some months as a combination of drugs

- Side effects of both endocrine and chemotherapy can be challenging, but management of these is continually improving

Drug treatments

Surgery and radiotherapy treat the breast cancer in the breast and associated lymph nodes. For some patients with early breast cancer, this may not be enough, as the disease is at significant risk of recurring and spreading elsewhere. This is because 'rogue' cancer cells may have escaped to other parts of the body through the lymphatic or blood circulation, and therefore a local treatment approach to the breast alone would be insufficient to prevent a tumour recurrence. Drug treatments, otherwise known as systemic therapies, enter the circulation and potentially target these rogue cells, thereby reducing the risk of a breast cancer recurrence. These treatments are however associated with a range of side effects, which can be significant for the patient. Most women with invasive breast cancer will have drug therapies included as a part of their treatment plan. The main exceptions are women who have other medical conditions or whose age makes it unlikely that they will tolerate the side effects, or women whose tumours are very small, where the potential benefits of treatment which are correspondingly small, do not outweigh the side effects. Systemic therapy may be given before (otherwise known as preoperative or neoadjuvant therapy) or after surgery (otherwise known as adjuvant therapy) is performed.

Preoperative versus postoperative systemic therapy

As discussed briefly in Chapter 6, the traditional approach for most patients with early breast cancer (i.e. cancer confined to the breast and/or lymph nodes) is to have the surgery first. This will both remove the cancer and allow more information about the tumour from the pathologist's assessment of the excised tumour. Preoperative or neoadjuvant therapy is when systemic treatment is given before surgery, and is usually chemotherapy and HER2-directed therapy, but can also include endocrine therapy. The advantage of this approach is that for women with larger tumours, and for patients with triple negative and HER2-positive subtypes of breast cancer, where it is highly likely they will need chemotherapy anyway after surgery, the drugs may make the tumour shrink and potentially eradicate the tumour completely. Patients who have a complete response have an extremely good prognosis. This approach also allows for a smaller and potentially more effective operation. It also means that both the patient and the doctor can actually measure if the drugs are working on the tumour by watching it shrink.

Endocrine therapy

Most breast cancers grow under the influence of circulating hormones, most notably oestrogen. Endocrine treatment options that target the hormone-responsive nature of breast cancer have advanced our ability to successfully combat and cure these cancers in patients whose tumours express the ER and/or PR, which constitute about two-thirds of all breast cancers. Like chemotherapy, endocrine therapy is a form of systemic, or full body, treatment.

Endocrine treatments work by either reducing the overall amount of oestrogen in the body or by stopping the oestrogen present exerting its usual effect. The result for hormone-responsive breast cancer cells is that they are starved of the oestrogen they require to help them grow. These therapies include tamoxifen, aromatase inhibitors (anastrazole, letrozole, and exemestane), and drugs that suppress the ovarian production of oestrogen by acting on the pituitary gland. Endocrine therapies are effective in both early stage and metastatic breast cancer, and are in general preferred to chemotherapy in hormone-receptor-positive breast cancer due to better efficacy (i.e. they are very good at targeting these cancer cells), ease of administration (i.e. a tablet a day rather than injected drugs), and relatively better side effect profile.

Other, non-cancerous body tissues may miss out on the beneficial effect of oestrogen due to the cancer treatment, leading to not so desirable effects, for example, the potential to make bone thinning or osteoporosis worse by aromatase inhibitors. While hormonal treatments are easier in general for patients to tolerate than chemotherapy, there are still some significant side effects that need to be considered. This is particularly important given that hormonal treatment is usually given over a long duration (5–10 years). The most common side effects women may experience with endocrine therapies are symptoms similar to those of menopause, such as hot flushes, sweats, mood and sleep disturbance, reduced interest in sex, and vaginal dryness. Women still having menstrual periods may notice a change in their cycle or even a complete stop of menstruation. Symptoms are usually at their worst when treatment is first started and often settle down within weeks to months. For women who do not tolerate these side effects, there may be other therapies that can be given to manage some of these, such as low dose antidepressant medication. Sometimes switching from one type of endocrine therapy to another is very helpful.

Tamoxifen

The primary source of oestrogen in pre- and perimenopausal women (before and around menopause) is the ovaries. Tamoxifen is recommended for premenopausal women with hormone-receptor-positive cancers, but is also a treatment option for postmenopausal women. Tamoxifen is a tablet taken once daily, for between 5 and 10 years' duration. It is transported in the bloodstream and binds onto the ERs in breast cancer cells, interrupting the effects of circulating oestrogens in the cancer cells. It does not affect oestrogen production and circulating levels. It has been successfully used to treat breast cancer for over 40 years and is associated with a reduction of breast cancer recurrence by about half.

The common menopausal side effects have just been discussed. In addition, tamoxifen can stimulate growth of the uterine (womb) lining. Occasionally, women may experience abnormal vaginal bleeding as a result. In rare situations, if left unchecked, there is a small increased risk of uterine cancer. It has been estimated that for women on tamoxifen, the additional risk of developing uterine cancer beyond that for other women equates to about 1 in 1,000 per year. There is also a very small increased risk of blood clots such as deep venous thrombosis in the legs, pelvis, and lungs. Compared to the potentially large benefit of treating their breast cancer, most women find these unlikely side effects an acceptable risk.

Ovarian suppression and ablation

Another endocrine treatment option for pre- and perimenopausal women is the shutting down of the ovarian production of oestrogen. This would essentially convert the patient into a postmenopausal state, bringing with it complications of early menopause. It is thus not routinely recommended to all patients with hormone-receptor-positive breast cancer, but considered in women with higher-risk breast cancer where a more aggressive therapeutic approach is required. It has also been shown to be beneficial in reducing the risk of breast cancer recurrence in some patients with triple negative (ER-, PR-, and HER2-negative) tumours. This may be achieved with medication to temporarily stop the ovaries making oestrogen, or surgical removal of the ovaries or occasionally by radiotherapy to the ovaries. It is only relevant in premenopausal women, as the ovaries in postmenopausal women no longer produce oestrogen.

The most commonly used class of drugs for this purpose is gonadotrophin-releasing hormone analogues (GnRH analogues), such as goserelin (Zoladex) and triptorelin. GnRH analogues trick the pituitary gland into reducing production of luteinizing hormone (LH), which is required by the ovaries to drive oestrogen production. A drug-induced lack of LH puts the ovaries to 'sleep'—a temporary menopause—while the drug is in use. Goserelin is usually administered monthly by an injection under the skin. Ovarian ablation refers to the permanent shutting down of the ovaries. This can be achieved by surgical removal of the ovaries or by radiotherapy to the ovaries. Some women prefer this to repeated monthly injections. There may also be some additional benefit in surgical removal of the ovaries in some women who have a family history of breast or ovarian cancer as they may be at an increased risk of developing ovarian cancer themselves.

Induced early menopause will be associated with temporary or permanent loss of fertility, predisposition to osteoporosis, and other long-term effects. These issues will be addressed later in this book in Chapter 10. The sudden reduction in oestrogen levels after ovarian ablation (see Table 8.1) can bring on quite severe menopausal symptoms. Usually, these will settle down in time.

Table 8.1 Comparison of removing ovaries versus using drugs to suppress ovarian function

Ovarian ablation	Ovarian suppression
Permanent menopause	Usually temporary menopause
Permanent loss of fertility	Fertility may return
One treatment only	Monthly injections for 2–5 years
Removes the risk of developing ovarian cancer	May decrease the risk of developing ovarian cancer

Goserelin or other ovarian suppression drugs are also sometimes used during chemotherapy in women keen to preserve their fertility as they shut the ovaries down and essentially allow them to 'sleep' during the administration of chemotherapy, which is toxic to a functioning ovary and destroys the developing eggs within it.

Aromatase inhibitors

While tamoxifen acts directly on the ER in cancer cells and remains a treatment option in postmenopausal women, another class of endocrine therapy called aromatase inhibitors may also be used, which are slightly more effective, and has a different side effect profile.

The ovaries in postmenopausal women are not producing oestrogen, however, all of us will have some oestrogen produced in our bodies. The main source of circulating oestrogen in older women is body fat where the enzyme aromatase converts other hormones to oestrogen. This process can be blocked by a class of drugs called aromatase inhibitors. These include letrozole (Femara), anastrazole (Arimidex), and exemestane (Aromasin). These drugs inactivate aromatase, thus stopping the conversion of adrenal gland hormones into oestrogen in the fat tissue. In contrast to tamoxifen, which blocks oestrogen binding to hormone receptors in breast cancer cells, aromatase inhibitors aim to reduce the total amount of oestrogen circulating in the body. This class of drugs is not used in pre- and perimenopausal women as the drug itself can stimulate oestrogen production in functioning ovaries. Like tamoxifen, they are tablets that are given once daily for 5–10 years, and reduce the incidence of recurrence by about half.

In addition to the common menopausal side effects just discussed, there are some specific side effects associated with aromatase inhibitors. Aromatase

Table 8.2 Comparison of tamoxifen versus aromatase inhibitors

	Tamoxifen	Aromatase inhibitors
Indication	Women of all menopausal status	Postmenopausal women
Benefits	Reduces incidence of breast cancer recurrence by about half	Reduces incidence of breast cancer recurrence by about half
Drawbacks	Menopausal symptoms Small risk of blood clots Possible irregular vaginal bleeding Small risk of womb cancer	Menopausal symptoms May develop joint pains Increased risk of osteoporosis and bone fractures with long-term use

inhibitors can cause joint pain, in particular affecting the small joints of the hands and feet. In some women, these pains can be quite difficult to treat although there are various strategies used to deal with the problem including simple pain medications or anti-inflammatory gels. The incidence of osteoporosis and bone fractures is also increased in women on these drugs. Thus, a baseline bone mineral density scan as well as annual monitoring is recommended. Patients on aromatase inhibitors are also advised to take vitamin D supplementation, ensure adequate calcium intake, and participate in weight-bearing exercises (see Table 8.2).

Bone modifying agents

More recently, bisphosphonates, a class of drugs used to treat osteoporosis, were found to reduce the rate of bone loss, as well as breast cancer recurrence in the bone, and improve survival in post-menopausal patients with early stage breast cancer. This includes patients with natural menopause or those induced by ovarian suppression or ablation. Bisphosphonate drugs include zoledronic acid (Zoladex), which is given intravenously every 6 months, or clodronate, a tablet taken every day. Another type of bone modifying therapy, denosumab (Prolia), had similar benefits, although long-term survival data is still pending.

HER2-directed therapies

Around 15–20% of breast cancers make an excess of a protein called the HER2 growth factor receptor on the cell surface. This results in an abnormal signal that stimulates these cells to grow and invade. Cancer cells that overexpress HER2 are also referred to as 'HER2-positive' or 'HER2-amplified'. HER2-positive tumours have poorer outcomes compared to HER2-negative tumours. However, with the development of effective therapies that target HER2, the prognosis or outlook of patients with this subtype of breast cancer has improved significantly. This class of therapy may be used in early breast cancer in the preoperative (neoadjuvant) setting or following surgery (adjuvant), and in metastatic breast cancer, and is typically given in combination with chemotherapy.

Trastuzumab (Herceptin)

The drug trastuzumab (more commonly known as Herceptin) is an antibody that attaches specifically to HER2, and turns off the strong HER2 signals which are making the cells grow. This drug is only effective in the tumours that overexpress HER2—that is, have abnormal amounts of the growth signaller. Clinical trials have shown that for women whose tumours have this abnormal amount of HER2, trastuzumab in combination with chemotherapy will improve the chance that cancer will not return by about a third. It is administered every three weeks by intravenous or subcutaneous injection for a year. Some women will experience mild flu-like symptoms initially, but overall it is very well tolerated. A small proportion of women can develop heart problems and it is routine to monitor the heart function by imaging every three to four months while on treatment. Should the heart function be affected, it may be managed by the addition of medications to improve heart function and by temporarily stopping trastuzumab. Some patients may not be able to recommence treatment with trastuzumab.

In the past, a full course of chemotherapy was recommended in combination with trastuzumab in early stage breast cancer. However, more recently, it has been demonstrated that for women with lower risk HER2-positive breast cancers (small tumours that have not spread to the lymph nodes), a shorter course of chemotherapy in combination with trastuzumab results in very good outcomes, with fewer side effects.

Pertuzumab (Perjeta)

Pertuzumab is newer class of antibody drug that targets a different portion of the HER2 protein. It is very similar to trastuzumab in its mode of action, and is used in combination with trastuzumab and chemotherapy. Like trastuzumab, it is given every 3 weeks, but only intravenously. In addition to the risk of cardiac side effects and flu-like symptoms, it is also associated with diarrhoea, which can be managed with the use of medication. Currently, the clinical trial data demonstrating its efficacy is only in the preoperative (neoadjuvant) setting for early stage breast cancer and in patients with metastatic breast cancer, where it seems to be quite a bit better than trastuzumab alone. We expect results of its use in the postoperative (adjuvant) setting in the near future.

Neratinib (Nerlynx)

More recently, in 2017, the Food and Drug Administration (FDA) in the United States approved neratinib for use to prevent recurrence in patients with early stage HER2-positive breast cancer who have finished at least one year of trastuzumab therapy. The benefit of one year of neratinib, which comes in the form of a tablet, was found primarily in women with ER-positive and HER2-positive breast cancer. It is associated with a high incidence of diarrhoea as a side effect. This is not currently funded for use outside the United States.

Chemotherapy

Chemotherapy is drug treatment given usually via a vein into the bloodstream. These drugs target cells by several different mechanisms, resulting in cell death. Although both normal cells and cancer cells are affected by chemotherapy, most normal body cells are much better able to recover (or are more resistant) compared to cancer cells, giving rise to a what is called a therapeutic window—that is, a dose has been worked out that kills the cancer cells, but allows normal cells to recover. Chemotherapy is given over several cycles, each round resulting in the death of more cancer cells. This also allows for the normal cells in the body to recover in between. The normal cells that are most affected are those with a rapid turnover, such as hair follicle cells (hence hair loss) and in the bone marrow where blood cells are made (hence some of the other complications such as anaemia and low white cell and platelet counts). Some of the more serious side effects, such as a suppression of the immune system, can be life-threatening, thus a decision to proceed with chemotherapy, particularly in patients who are not fit, needs to be carefully considered.

Chemotherapy is most often given after surgery to the breast and axilla but before radiotherapy or hormone therapy, if these are required. This is called adjuvant chemotherapy. It may also be given preoperatively as neoadjuvant chemotherapy. This is most commonly when the tumour is large in relation to the breast (locally advanced breast cancer) and the aim of the chemotherapy is to shrink the tumour, thus possibly allowing breast-conserving surgery. In some women the tumour is not amenable to surgery when they are first diagnosed (because the tumour is stuck to the chest wall or of an inflammatory type), so the chemotherapy is aimed at making surgery by mastectomy possible.

Chemotherapy reduces the chance of cancer recurring by about a third in early breast cancer. It is effective in all breast cancer subtypes; however, it is not always necessary, and is a decision based upon the risks and presumed benefits of chemotherapy. The decision by the cancer team to recommend chemotherapy depends on several factors:

- How aggressive the patient's tumour appears clinically and following patho-
  logical assessment (the tumour stage)

- How much the tumour is likely to respond to treatments other than chemotherapy (such as endocrine therapy, which is generally better tolerated and
  more effective than chemotherapy in hormone-receptor-positive breast
  cancer)

- A patient's age and whether the woman herself is fit enough to undergo
  chemotherapy

- The choice of the patient based on the risks and benefits, and personal views

The benefits of chemotherapy have been worked out from information gained
from large clinical trials for which the patients have agreed to enter a study
where two treatment regimens are compared for effectiveness on the cancer
and side effects. Most chemotherapy treatment for early stage breast cancer
consists of a combination of drugs, either given together, or one after another.
The actual combination given to an individual woman will depend on many
factors, including: the type of breast cancer; the age and fitness of the patient; the side effect profile of the drugs; the experience and preferences of
the treating oncologist; and the cost and the availability within the hospital
prescribing system.s

The most common classes of chemotherapy drugs prescribed for early stage
breast cancer contain either an anthracycline drug, such as doxorubicin
(Adriamycin) and epirubicin; and/or a taxane, such as paclitaxel (Taxol), and
docetaxel (Taxotere). These are the two most effective classes of chemotherapy
used in breast cancer. A patient needs to discuss this in detail with her medical
oncologist to fully understand the decisions made and her potential side effects
and benefits. In patients who receive preoperative chemotherapy and have residual cancer at the time of surgery, six to eight cycles of capecitabine (Xeloda),
which is a different class of chemotherapy, have been shown to reduce the risk
of breast cancer recurrence. The benefit is primarily seen in patients with triple
negative (ER-, PR-, and HER2-negative) tumours.

Chemotherapy is usually prescribed and supervised by a specialist medical oncologist. Treatment is usually in a specialist chemotherapy day treatment unit.
Blood tests prior to treatment ensure that the bone marrow has recovered from
the previous cycle of chemotherapy, and the other organs such as the liver and
kidney are functioning normally. Chemotherapy nurses who administer the
drugs are also an invaluable source of information and help with managing
side effects. Chemotherapy is given in 'cycles': a day of the chemotherapy treatment followed by a period of no treatment to allow the body time to recover,
prior to another dose of chemotherapy. This will typically last for between three

and six months. Sometimes, cycles may be compressed from 3 to 2 weeks, otherwise known as dose-dense chemotherapy. While this has been shown to improve outcomes slightly, it is typically only offered to younger patients, as there is a shorter time allowed for the patient to recover from the previous cycle of chemotherapy, and also associated with an increased risk of bone marrow toxicity.

Virtually all patients receiving chemotherapy will experience some side effects, although for many these will be tolerable, and many women can continue to work and do regular exercise. Some patients diagnosed with breast cancer during pregnancy may even continue their pregnancy through chemotherapy. Common side effects of chemotherapy include fatigue, nausea, a sore mouth, and hair loss. It is difficult to predict who will get side effects and to what extent, and it may vary over the course of the treatments. Any side effects, even mild ones, should be reported to the nursing and medical teams as most can be managed very well. A major breakthrough in cancer care has been the improved therapies used to prevent and treat nausea, and these treatments constitute an integral part of chemotherapy management.

Scalp cooling is an option for some women on some of the less intensive chemotherapy regimens as a way to try to reduce hair loss. This involves wearing a cold cap filled with coolant during the chemotherapy infusion for a few hours, which works by bringing the scalp temperature down to 4°C, and thereby causing the blood vessels to constrict, and reducing the chemotherapy effect on the hair follicles. This does not work in the setting of more intensive chemotherapy regimens, and works a lot less well in people with some hair types such as Afro-American hair.

Chemotherapy often causes early menopause, and subsequent loss of fertility in premenopausal women and is discussed in detail in Chapter 12. It is important that fertility be discussed with the treating team as soon as possible after diagnosis, and some patients may want to have their eggs collected and stored for future use prior to starting chemotherapy. GnRH agonists such as goserelin are sometimes given with chemotherapy in an attempt to protect the ovaries, and hence a woman's fertility, from the chemotherapy effects.

📄 Case study

Lisa was 44 when she found a lump in her right breast. At first she thought it may be lumpiness associated with her period, as it was rather tender. But it persisted over two cycles, so she went to her GP who urgently ordered an ultrasound and mammogram and a needle biopsy. This showed a cancer and both the examination and imaging suggested it was about 2 cm in size.

Lisa had a lumpectomy and sentinel node biopsy and the tumour was found to be just over 2 cm (22 mm) in size, and a grade 2 ductal cancer which had not spread to her lymph nodes. The tumour was hormone-receptor-positive and HER2-negative.

She discussed further treatment with both her surgeon and a medical and radiation oncologist. They informed Lisa that her case had been discussed in their multidisciplinary meeting and the team suggested she should consider chemotherapy, radiotherapy, and hormone therapy. Although it was likely Lisa would suffer some side effects of chemotherapy including fatigue and nausea, however, the oncologist reassured her that these symptoms could be helped with both some drugs and a healthy lifestyle including exercise. However, she was likely to lose her hair (on her head, pubic region, and possibly eyebrows) during treatment with chemotherapy and her local hospital did not have access to cold caps which can help lessen this.

Lisa was very worried about the chemotherapy and scared she would not be able to tolerate it. She discussed this with her family and the breast care nurse arranged for her to meet another patient who had gone through treatment.

She also understood from her oncologist that the chemotherapy would improve the chance of her breast cancer not coming back. If she had NO further systemic treatment (so only surgery and radiotherapy) the chance of tumour recurring would be around 35%. With the addition of just the hormone drug tamoxifen, this improved to only 25% of women ever getting cancer back but with chemotherapy as well only 15% of women will ever have the cancer recurring.

Lisa decided to go for the chemotherapy and was surprised how well she coped. She had to take time off work for a few days after each chemotherapy treatment, but found joining an exercise programme run by a local cancer support group, and eating a healthy diet meant she got back to perhaps 80% of normal in between treatments.

She had a setback on the fifth cycle of chemotherapy, when she developed a very low white cell count and a chest infection which needed treatment for 3 days in hospital, but adjusting her drugs meant this did not happen on the sixth and final cycle.

Lisa completed radiotherapy 10 weeks after the end of chemotherapy—it took over 9 months for all the acute treatment to finish, and then she went on to tamoxifen which would be for at least 5 years.

Further resources

Macmillan Cancer Support. Changes to appearance and body image. Available at: https://www.macmillan.org.uk/information-and-support/coping/changes-to-appearance-and-body-image/dealing-with-hair-lossPREDICT. Available at: https://predict.nhs.uk/

PREDICT. Available at: https://predict.nhs.uk/

9

Treating special types of breast cancer

 Key points

- There is a wide spectrum of different breast cancers presenting unique challenges

- Proper understanding of breast cancer type is crucial in maximizing treatment efficacy

- Preinvasive breast cancers are confined to the breast, whereas invasive cancers can spread elsewhere

- Breast cancer treatment is tailored to a particular cancer in a particular patient

- Men get breast cancer too—albeit rarely!

Ductal carcinoma in situ (DCIS)

DCIS is an early type of breast cancer, which by definition is confined to the milk ducts in the breast and thus cannot spread to lymph nodes or other parts of the body.

The cells under the microscope have features of cancer cells and it is likely that several changes have occurred in the genes within the cells, which makes them act somewhat like cancer—that is, they have lost some of the checks on their growth and division and can spread down ducts. This in itself would not be important if they stayed at this stage. However, some DCIS will go on to become an invasive cancer which can then spread into the breast and other parts of the body and ultimately harm the patient.

DCIS comes in several types and is defined by features of the cells themselves which reflect how quickly they are growing and how likely they are to progress to an actual breast cancer. These are called low and intermediate grade (or low-risk DCIS) and high-grade DCIS. Like invasive cancer, DCIS can also have receptors on the cells for hormones and the growth factor HER2, although as these treatments are not often used in DCIS the pathologist may not measure these receptors nor report on them.

DCIS is most commonly a condition that does not produce any symptoms, although occasionally it can form a lump or cause a blood-stained discharge from the nipple. It is usually found on a routine mammogram, or a mammogram done for another symptom, and can show up as a cluster or line of white dots called microcalcification (see Fig. 9.1).

Low-grade DCIS is often a chance finding on biopsy, or can be just a shadow or calcifications on a mammogram. Small areas of low-grade DCIS (less than 2 or 3 cm) are usually considered at very low risk of becoming cancer and are treated just with local surgery. In fact, several studies around the world are looking to see if they can simply be watched with no active treatment.

Higher-grade DCIS, and in particular that which is extensive over more than a few centimetres, and has HER2 receptors, is much more likely to become an invasive cancer so needs complete removal, which in some instances is by mastectomy. If the breast is conserved, radiotherapy is usually recommended for most high-grade and some lower-grade DCIS. If a high-grade DCIS does

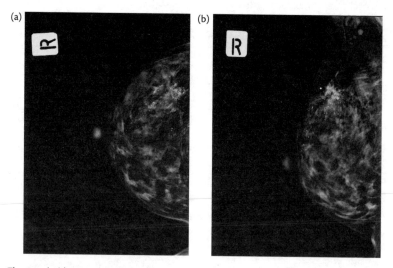

Fig. 9.1 (a, b) Microcalcification in ductal carcinoma *in situ* (DCIS).

come back it is likely to be as a high-grade so more aggressive invasive cancer, so complete treatment is important.

The place of drug treatment in DCIS is controversial, and endocrine treatments such as Tamoxifen may be suggested to prevent a second area of DCIS or invasive cancer developing.

Lobular carcinoma *in situ* (LCIS)

LCIS is a non-invasive neoplastic process, similar in some ways to DCIS but with two important differences. Firstly, where DCIS is a cancerous change formed within and confined to the milk ducts, LCIS is a multiplication of abnormal cells from the lining of the breast lobules, where milk is produced. Secondly, like DCIS, LCIS indicates an increased risk of invasive breast cancer, but unlike DCIS, surgical removal of LCIS does not, in most cases, reduce the risk of invasive cancer as the risk is not confined to one area, but is across both breasts. In fact, LCIS indicates an 8–10 times increase in relative risk for developing invasive breast cancer in either breast. This is probably due to the propensity for LCIS to be multifocal and/or bilateral.

LCIS has no typical clinical or radiological features. As such, it is usually an incidental or chance finding in a needle biopsy or surgical excision specimen. Proper management in such situations depends on both the perceived risk of any concurrent undetected cancer and appropriate surveillance and/or risk reduction strategies to counter the increased possibility of a future breast cancer.

Most LCIS found on needle biopsy is 'classic' in type. In the absence of any other finding triggering surgical excision, and assuming the radiological changes which led to the needle biopsy in the first place have been explained, surveillance with annual breast imaging may be quite reasonable. Some subtypes of LCIS—most notably 'pleomorphic LCIS'—behave more like DCIS. That is, they have a higher tendency for progression to invasive cancer. Wide local excision and adjuvant radiotherapy (or mastectomy) is usually recommended.

Women with LCIS face an annual incidence for breast cancer of between 1 and 2%. This is similar to the risk associated with a strong family history of breast cancer. Medical review and annual surveillance imaging with a combination of mammogram, ultrasound, and sometimes MRI is generally recommended.

Risk reduction strategies include medication and surgery. Drugs such as tamoxifen and aromatase inhibitors taken for 5 years will roughly halve the risk of breast cancer. This benefit needs to be weighed against the medication risks and side effects. In addition, and compared with proper surveillance imaging, drug prophylaxis may not improve overall prognosis.

Prophylactic mastectomy is an extreme option that is usually not recommended but may be appropriate in some women after careful consideration and within the confines of a multidisciplinary team plan.

Lobular breast cancer

Lobular breast cancer comprises approximately 10% of all breast cancer. It most often expresses the hormone receptors only, although it can uncommonly be HER2-positive or a triple negative breast cancer subtype. It is characterized by the absence of the E-cadherin protein. Lobular breast cancers are defined by the way they grow, which is typically described as in an Indian file, or a line, as opposed to clusters of cells making a defined lump. As such, lobular cancers can sometimes span a much larger area than the average invasive ductal breast cancer. They can also be more difficult to detect as the lump in the breast can be ill-defined and harder to feel, and mammograms and ultrasounds are not always as accurate in detecting these cancers. It can also potentially metastasize to unusual parts of the body, including the meninges, which line the brain, and the peritoneum, which lines the abdomen. Treatment is not dissimilar to ductal cancers and depends on the expression of hormone receptors and HER2. There is some data that suggests that aromatase inhibitors may be relatively more beneficial than tamoxifen in the adjuvant treatment of lobular breast cancers relative to ductal cancers.

Locally advanced breast cancer

Locally advanced breast cancer is a type of breast cancer that involves surrounding structures, are typically large, and found more often in patients who have presented or have been diagnosed late. Involved surrounding structures can include the skin of the breast, where it can cause an ulcer and bleeding, or the tumour can become fixed to underlying muscles. Lymph nodes can also be fixed to surrounding tissues in locally advanced breast cancer. The term *locally advanced* can also be used just to mean the tumour is large (more than 5 cm in size).

Locally advanced breast cancer is often treated with preoperative chemotherapy or sometimes endocrine therapy, to downstage the cancer, followed almost always by surgery and radiotherapy. Modern drug treatments will often shrink locally advanced tumours down to a size where breast-conserving surgery is possible. The aim of treatment in locally advanced cancer is the same as with early breast cancer: to cure the disease. The chance of cancer coming back is significantly higher than with smaller cancers, and treatment usually more extensive, but the cure rate has improved greatly in recent years. Most patients will do very well, and many will be cured.

Inflammatory breast cancer

Around 2% of patients will have a diagnosis of an inflammatory cancer. This presents as a red breast with thickened dimpled skin (known as peau d'orange or orange peel, see Fig. 9.2), and sometimes but not always a discrete mass. The appearance is because the cancer has infiltrated the tiny lymphatic vessels under the skin blocking drainage of tissue fluid and causing an inflamed looking appearance. In fact, some women may have been treated with antibiotics in the mistaken belief that it was a case of mastitis (breast infection).

Suspected inflammatory cancer always needs a mammogram and biopsy and because it is known to be an aggressive form of breast cancer, it is important to undertake tests of the whole patient (usually a computed tomography (CT) scan and bone scan or positron-emission tomography (PET) scan and blood tests) to ensure there is no spread to other organs at diagnosis.

If the cancer is limited to the breast and/or lymph nodes, it is best to start treatment with chemotherapy as an operation, even a mastectomy, before chemotherapy can leave behind small amounts of cancer in the skin. After chemotherapy a mastectomy is needed to ensure all tumour is removed (even if the chemotherapy response seems very good, small amounts of tumour are often left but cannot be seen) and removal of lymph nodes in the axilla. Sentinel

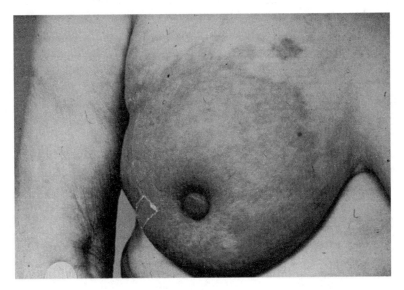

Fig. 9.2 Inflammatory breast cancer.

node biopsy is controversial in inflammatory cancer as it is not very accurate in detecting where the lowest node lies, so many patients will be recommended to have a full axillary clearance. Reconstruction is an option but needs careful discussion within the multidisciplinary team and with the patient.

After surgery radiotherapy to the chest wall is also recommended, and often the lymph node area.

Close follow-up is then undertaken. Unfortunately, recurrence is not uncommon (see Chapter 12 on advanced disease).

Breast cancer in men

Breast cancer can occur in men but is uncommon—less than 1% of breast cancers are in men and in most countries no more than a few hundred men each year are diagnosed. It usually affects older men and occurs more often in families which carry a high-risk gene fault—the *BRCA2* gene.

Like in women, the cancer usually presents as a lump or nipple change. Breast swelling in men can also be due to a benign condition called gynaecomastia, but any change should be reported to a doctor. Investigations are the same as in women, as both a mammogram and ultrasound can be performed, as can a needle biopsy. Treatment is usually by mastectomy and all male breast cancers have hormone receptors, so hormone treatment with Tamoxifen will be recommended, plus or minus chemotherapy and radiotherapy.

Because breast cancer is traditionally seen as a woman's cancer, men may feel reluctant to talk about it and to seek support. Good information and resources are listed next and detail how breast nurses are trained to care for men with breast cancer and their families, too.

📄 Case studies
Inflammatory breast cancer

Catherine is a 52-year-old teacher who had noted an area of redness in her left breast for at least 4 months. She has initially thought this was an infection after a mosquito bite to her breast while on summer holidays and indeed had received a course of antibiotics for 2 weeks from her general practitioner for this. However, the area of redness did not get better and she noted her whole breast felt quite swollen and heavy. Her husband urged her to return to her GP to find out what was causing this.

Her GP was also concerned so referred her to the local hospital's breast clinic, where she was seen by a breast surgeon and breast nurse 1 week later. They explained they were concerned this was a kind of cancer called an inflammatory breast cancer and so she underwent a mammogram and ultrasound which showed no actual mass in the breast but thickened skin and enlarged lymph nodes under the arm. A biopsy of the lymph nodes and a small biopsy of the thickened skin and underlying tissue showed this was a triple negative breast cancer. She had a CT scan of her chest, abdomen, and pelvis, and a bone scan which were normal. She also had an MRI scan of her breast and a PET scan that showed that the involved areas were limited to her breast and her axillary lymph nodes.

The following week Catherine saw a medical oncologist and after some more tests started preoperative chemotherapy. The redness and swelling went away completely within 2 months, and the lymph nodes shrank on ultrasound, although they remained a little larger than normal.

About 6 weeks after the completion of chemotherapy, she underwent a total mastectomy and had lymph nodes removed from under her arm. She did not have reconstruction at the time as both she and her doctors were keen for her to start radiotherapy about 3 weeks after surgery, although she keen to consider this after all other treatments were finished.

The pathology report from her operation showed that the tumour had almost completely disappeared with only a residual area of DCIS left behind, and there was no tumour found in her lymph nodes. In fact, three nodes looked like they had previously had tumour in them which had been eliminated by the chemotherapy. Fortunately, she needed no other treatment.

Six months after the end of all treatment she had a mammogram of her right breast, which was normal and a repeat CT and bone scan that confirmed she had no recurrent disease, so she went on to have a left breast reconstruction.

Male breast cancer

Jim is a 72-year-old retired widower who while playing golf noticed his arm brush against a hard lump in his left breast. He mentioned this to his golf partner who suggested he get it checked out as he had heard a recent media campaign saying that men can get breast cancer too. Jim thought this was pretty unlikely—he had never heard of breast cancer in men and there was none in his family. However, he also mentioned it to his daughter who stressed he should go and visit his doctor.

His doctor explained that while some breast lumps were just swellings of breast tissue it was important to do some tests to see what was causing it. This included first a clinical examination of his whole body, some blood tests, and a chest X-ray, all of which were normal. The GP then referred him to a breast surgeon who arranged a mammogram, ultrasound, and needle biopsy, which confirmed a breast cancer.

Jim underwent a mastectomy and sentinel node biopsy which showed a 2 cm cancer with no lymph nodes involved. Like all breast cancers in men it was strongly ER and PR positive (that is sensitive to female hormones) so Jim started on the drug tamoxifen for 5 years, and had check-ups with the surgeon every 6 months, but was soon back to playing golf, and recovered very well.

Further resources

Breast Cancer Network Australia. *Breast Cancer in Men*. Available at: https://www.bcna.org.au/understanding-breast-cancer/breast-cancer-in-men/

Cancer Australia. *Ductal Carcinoma in Situ*. Available at: https://breast-cancer.canceraustralia.gov.au/types/ductal-carcinoma-situ

NIH National Cancer Institute. *Inflammatory Breast Cancer*. Available at: https://www.cancer.gov/types/breast/ibc-fact-sheet

Triple Negative Breast Cancer Foundation. *Understanding Triple Negative Breast Cancer*. Available at: https://tnbcfoundation.org/understanding-triple-negative-breast-cancer/

10

Surviving and thriving

> ## ➔ Key points
>
> ◆ Chemotherapy decreases fertility—this should be considered prior to starting chemotherapy in women who have not completed their family
>
> ◆ Cool caps can halve hair loss during chemotherapy
>
> ◆ Many breast cancer drug treatments will cause menopause symptoms, including loss of sex drive, but there are strategies available to help with these
>
> ◆ Women on treatment for breast cancer should consider having bone density measurements
>
> ◆ Fatigue is common with chemotherapy and regular exercise can help
>
> ◆ Depression will affect up to 30% of women after cancer and can be managed if recognized
>
> ◆ Weight gain is a common complaint—a healthy diet and exercise are the best remedies
>
> ◆ Lymphoedema occurs in some women after axillary surgery; physiotherapy can help prevent and treat it
>
> ◆ Let your oncologist know about any complementary therapies you are using

Fertility

For young women who have not yet completed their family and are diagnosed with breast cancer, this can seem like a double blow. Chemotherapy agents will 'age' the ovaries by about 10 years, meaning that for many they will struggle with trying to conceive a child in the future and may become menopausal. If this is of concern to the patient, it is important that they are referred as soon as possible to a fertility specialist to discuss options. Preferably this should be before starting chemotherapy.

After assessment (which often includes blood tests, an ultrasound of the ovaries, and sometimes even a sperm test of the male partner) the fertility specialist may discuss options for a cycle of *in vitro* fertilization (IVF) prior to chemotherapy to allow embryo or egg storage, or the newer and less proven ovarian tissue storage. These may not be covered by government or health insurer funding. There is no evidence that these are dangerous in terms of the breast cancer as long as treatment is not delayed too long.

Options also exist to protect the ovaries during chemotherapy with drugs which temporarily shut them down (such as Goserelin or Zoladex), which should be discussed by the oncologist before starting treatment.

After breast cancer, if on no drug treatment and the cancer has not returned, it does seem safe to consider a pregnancy if the woman wishes to. A current study (POSITIVE) is assessing if it is safe to consider this within a few years, interrupting endocrine therapy to do so.

Hair loss

Most chemotherapy agents cause hair loss—a very visible sign of cancer. The development of cool caps is helping some patients retain at least some (usually around 50%) of the hair. These are not available in all chemotherapy units and may be in great demand if they are. They work by cooling the scalp before and during chemotherapy to decrease the blood containing the drug that gets to the hair follicles, and shutting down hair follicle turnover at this time.

Menopause symptoms

Many women are around the age of the menopause (45–60) at diagnosis of breast cancer, and some will have been on hormone replacement therapy (HRT) which they are advised to stop. Others will go into menopause because of treatments such as chemotherapy and others will get menopausal treatment side effects from the hormonal treatments they are given for breast cancer. All this adds up to 60–80% of women diagnosed with cancer developing menopausal symptoms including hot flushes and night sweats, poor concentration and sleep, decreased sex drive and vaginal dryness, and for some, bone thinning (osteoporosis) and even cardiovascular problems.

Simple strategies can help some symptoms, such as relaxation strategies and avoiding possible hot flush triggers (e.g. alcohol or caffeine), but many women require specialist treatment. Generally, it is advisable not to use HRT after breast cancer, although vaginal oestrogen can be discussed with the oncologist if vaginal moisturizers and lubricants are not working. A range of non-hormone medications for hot flushes have been shown to have some benefit, and assessment by a specialist menopause clinic can be useful to explore these other medications.

Complementary treatments and over the counter medications have not been shown to be very effective, and some may contain agents that are not recommended after cancer so need to be discussed with the patient's cancer treatment team. More information and suggestions can be found in the resources section.

Bone health

Bone loss or osteoporosis is more common after breast cancer partly because it is associated with menopause, which may be precipitated early by breast cancer treatments. The drugs commonly used for oestrogen-receptor (ER) positive breast cancer called aromatase inhibitors (anastrazole, letrozole, and exemestane) all contribute to bone loss. It is very important to prevent bone loss and possible fractures as we age, so getting a bone density scan to check this is vital. Bone loss can be partly prevented by regular weight bearing exercise, not smoking, and decreasing alcohol, ensuring there is enough calcium in the diet and getting some sunshine so that vitamin D is made (15 minutes a day is recommended), but treatment with bone strengthening drugs may be needed.

Joint pains are another common side effect of the aromatase inhibitor drugs. These are probably due to very low oestrogen levels caused by these drugs. There is no one proven effective treatment, but simple anti-inflammatories may help, as may regular exercise. Changing to another drug can also often help, after discussion with the oncologist.

Fatigue

Fatigue is a common symptom of breast cancer and its treatment especially when undergoing chemotherapy. It is often associated with poor sleep patterns and mild depression. Ensuring a regular exercise regimen (although this can seem very hard if tired all the time), eating well, and sometimes short-term sleeping tablets can help.

Body image and sexuality

Surgery, especially mastectomy, and the side effects of other treatments can profoundly affect how a person feels about their body. This may improve with time and support of loved ones, but for some people this requires some specialist help from a psychologist—most breast units will have a specially trained psychologist who can help address these issues and help the woman feel better.

Sexuality is a complex issue, which is impacted by poor health generally—not surprisingly many people will feel less interested in sex during cancer treatment. However, for a very large proportion of women this issue continues to be a problem after active treatment has stopped and does not improve. It can be made worse by the effects of surgery on the body, by fatigue, and by depression. The anti-oestrogen treatments may cause vaginal dryness and other menopause symptoms which also affect sexual functioning. It is worth discussing these issues with the breast cancer doctor or nurse or general practitioner (GP). Referral to a sex therapist is also possible. More information is found in the 'Further resources' section.

Depression, anxiety, and grief

These feelings are common after breast cancer and in fact up to a third of women will develop some degree of depression or anxiety for a while after cancer. This is especially likely if a person has experienced this before—and we know one in five adults will have suffered from a mental health condition. Cancer can certainly cause this to recur or get worse. Depression is also more common in those that are socially isolated or have limited support networks, in younger women, and in those with more advanced disease.

Symptoms of anxiety include poor concentration, poor sleep, and persistent feelings of worry or unrest. Some will experience panic attacks. Symptoms of depression include persistent low mood, loss of interest in things normally found enjoyable, poor sleep, fatigue, and sometimes loss of appetite. Many of these symptoms are 'normal' during cancer treatment but if they are disrupting quality of life it is worth seeking help either from the GP or specialist or breast nurse. These symptoms can be helped by behavioural therapy and sometimes medication and seeing a psychologist can help.

Grief is a normal reaction to loss and change—losing a breast or losing the life we formally had can cause grief. However, many people do report that eventually they do learn to cope with their 'new normal' and many even derive strength from the adverse experience that is cancer and its treatment.

Weight change

One of the commonest complaints of women after breast cancer is that they have gained weight. Many women feel this is due to their medication. For most it can be attributed to changing diet and exercise or going into menopause. Changing medication is not likely to help, unfortunately—however, a good diet, cutting down alcohol, and exercise can. Many exercise and lifestyle programmes are now available in some countries for women after breast cancer and it is worth considering joining one of these as they have proven benefits in improving overall health and even in lowering a woman's chance of dying from other conditions such as heart disease.

Lymphoedema

Lymphoedema is swelling of the arm or breast after surgery and/or radiotherapy. Removal of some or all of the lymph glands under the arm can lead to this swelling in around one in five people, which can occur at any time after surgery. If the patient also has radiation therapy to the armpit it becomes even more likely. Fortunately, severe lymphoedema is such less common than many years ago, partly due to better surgery but also because of active physiotherapy intervention—both to educate patients on how to prevent it and also early and active treatment including compression garments and manual lymphatic drainage massage (see Fig. 10.1).

Rarely lymphoedema can occur even after sentinel node biopsy but is much less likely than after complete axillary clearance.

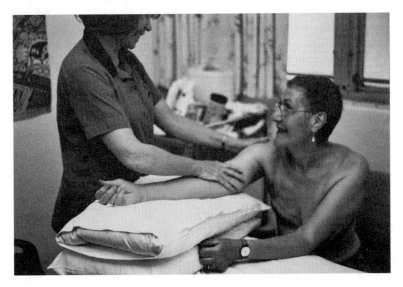

Fig. 10.1 A patient receiving lymphoedema treatment.

For severe lymphoedema, there is some good evidence that surgery to transplant the lymph nodes or channels can be effective.

More information on lymphoedema can be found in the 'Further resources' section.

Finances

Even in countries with universal healthcare, cancer is often a drain on household expenses due to loss of work, need to travel, or have help at home or with childcare, and incidental expenses of drug prescriptions and allied health such as physiotherapy. Private health cover often leaves patients with many out of pocket expenses, and several studies have added this up to many thousands of dollars for each year after cancer. Hospitals will have social work departments to which a patient can be referred for help with finances, including how to access government and charitable help schemes. Practical help with housework, for example, is often available through cancer charities and other local agencies.

Complementary treatments

A vast range of complementary treatments are available, some of which are very useful in improving quality of life or specific symptoms. Before embarking on what may be expensive and possibly useless and occasionally even harmful complementary treatment, it is worth researching it on some reputable websites. A recommended one follows next. It is also worth letting your oncologist know what you are using as a few complementary treatments may clash with some cancer drugs.

Thriving after breast cancer

Cancer diagnosis and treatment can be tough and lead to side effects and long-term health issues. But it is also an opportunity to re-evaluate the whole body's health. There is good evidence that doing regular exercise after breast cancer not only improves overall health but decreases the chance of cancer coming back. Many exercise programmes for people who have had cancer are available and provide tailored plans or gym classes with other cancer survivors, which many feel more comfortable with.

Maintaining a healthy weight also leads to a lower risk of cancer recurrence. The following list gives some tips on how to get and stay healthy after breast cancer.

Improving health after cancer

◆ Exercise for at least 150 minutes each week (enough to make you sweat or be somewhat short of breath)

◆ Keep weight healthy and body mass index (BMI) under 26

◆ Eat a healthy balanced diet with less sugar and red meat

◆ Moderate alcohol to less than two drinks per day

◆ Have regular screening for other cancers including bowel and cervical if appropriate

◆ Ensure your blood pressure and cholesterol are within normal limits—a check-up by the GP may be the best way to do this

◆ Stop smoking—if you smoke, this is the single most important thing you can ever do for your health

◆ Ensure you live a well-adjusted life that keeps you happy and motivated—a balance of work and play really is healthy!

Case study

Tammy underwent treatment for breast cancer 2 years ago, having a lumpectomy and radiotherapy, and is now on an aromatase inhibitor drug for 5 years. She was 57 when diagnosed and although considered herself to be fairly fit and well, she is a little overweight and has high blood pressure and diabetes on medication. Tammy had never done any formal exercise but kept busy in her job as a part-time retail assistant and looking after her two grandchildren aged 3 and 5.

She attended her 2-year check-up and was pleased to find the breast surgeon could find no new lumps or other breast problems and her mammogram was normal. However, she did confess that she had put on quite a bit of weight since her diagnosis and still had quite a few hot flushes since starting the medication and stopping the HRT she had been on before breast cancer.

Her doctor spent some time going through all of Tammy's health issues, and also suggested she discuss her health with her GP. Tammy was given some information about a local exercise class for women who had experienced cancer—she found going to this not only helped her feel fit and lose weight, which in fact improved her hot flushes and general well-being, but was also a good way to meet others who had similar experiences.

Further resources

Fertility

BIG Against Breast Cancer. *News*. Available at: http://www.breastinternationalgroup.org/news/ibcsg-positive-trial-set-investigate-pregnancy-after-breast-cancer/

Cancer Australia. *Managing Physical Changes Due to Breast Cancer*. Available at: https://canceraustralia.gov.au/affected-cancer/cancer-types/breast-cancer/living-breast-cancer/managing-physical-changes-due-breast-cancer/breast-cancer-and-fertility

Hair loss

Macmillan Cancer Support. *Coping with Hair Loss*. Available at: http://www.macmillan.org.uk/information-and-support/coping/side-effects-and-symptoms/hair-loss/scalp-cooling.html

Menopause

Cancer Australia. *Breast Cancer and Early Menopause: A Guide for Younger Women*. Available at: https://canceraustralia.gov.au/sites/default/files/publications/bcmc-breast-cancer-early-menopause-v2_504af03adb71c.pdf

The Royal Women's Hospital. *Menopause Symptoms After Cancer*. Available at: https://www.thewomens.org.au/patients-visitors/clinics-and-services/menopause/menopause-symptoms-after-cancer/

Sexuality

American Cancer Society. *Body Image and Sexuality After Breast Cancer*. Available at: https://www.cancer.org/cancer/breast-cancer/living-as-a-breast-cancer-survivor/body-image-and-sexuality-after-breast-cancer.html

Macmillan Cancer Support. *Relationships and Sex*. Available at: http://www.macmillan.org.uk/information-and-support/coping/relationships/your-sex-life-and-sexuality/index.html

Lymphoedema

Breastcancer.org. *Lymphedema*. Available at: http://www.breastcancer.org/treatment/lymphedema

Breast Cancer Network Australia. *Lymphoedema*. Available at: https://www.bcna.org.au/health-wellbeing/physical-wellbeing/lymphoedema/

Cancernet.uk. *Exercise and Breast Cancer*. Available at: http://www.cancernet.co.uk/ex-breast.htm

Complementary treatments

Memorial Sloan Kettering Cancer Center. *Integrative Medicine*. Available at: https://www.mskcc.org/cancer-care/diagnosis-treatment/symptom-management/integrative-medicine

Healthy living

Breast Cancer Network Australia. *Exercise and Breast Cancer*. Available at: https://www.bcna.org.au/media/2129/bcna_exercise_and_breast_cancer_booklet_0.pdf

Cancernet.co.uk. *Exercise and Cancer*. Available at: http://www.cancernet.co.uk/exercise.htm

WCA Encore. *Breast Cancer Exercise Program*. Available at: http://www.ywcaencore.org.au/

11

Follow-up

 Key points

♦ Follow-up physical examinations occur at least every 6 months after cancer

♦ Women should have an annual mammogram after cancer treatment, often with an ultrasound of the breast

♦ Other tests such as scans or blood tests done routinely are not of value

More than 80% of women will never develop a recurrence of their breast cancer. However, it is important to have regular checks both to ensure the cancer has not come back and to check that a new cancer has not developed. Early detection of recurrence, like early detection of the first cancer, means treatment is easier and more likely to be successful. Women who have had one breast cancer are somewhat more likely to develop another, so they require more regular screening for a new cancer—with an annual mammogram and sometimes ultrasound of the breasts. The chance of a second cancer is, however, still quite small, with less than 0.5% chance each year of a new cancer developing in the same breast or on the other side. As a woman gets older she 'uses up' some of this risk, so this figure gets even smaller. The only exceptions to this are women with familial cancer and known inherited gene faults (such as *BRCA1* and *2*) where she has up to 50% chance of getting a second cancer, prompting many of these women to consider bilateral mastectomy.

Specialist follow-up

Follow-up plans after breast cancer are very variable between hospitals, between doctors and between patients. Generally, a patient is seen after surgery by her surgeon. Depending on what other treatment she has will dictate which doctors arrange follow-up (which may be the surgeon, medical or radiation oncologist, or a combination of these), but generally a patient is seen every 6 months for 5 years and then often discharged from specialist care. These visits will include a breast examination, a mammogram, and often a breast ultrasound every year, a discussion of treatments and side effects, and an assessment of the general well-being of the person. Some units have instigated follow-up by other members of the team such as the breast nurses or breast physicians. In some sites, general practitioners (GPs) are becoming more involved with routine follow-up—a model known as 'shared care' where they see the patient either at all or some visits—but the key is to have a direct link into referring back to specialist care if problems arise, so these can be dealt with by experts in a timely manner.

X-rays and other tests

After a diagnosis of breast cancer, it is recommended to have a mammogram every year as the best interval to detect any recurrence or new cancer. Women with dense tissue on a mammogram (which makes it harder to detect cancer), or those where the first cancer was not seen on the mammogram, are recommended to also have an ultrasound. Occasionally in very young women or those with a strong family history of breast cancer, an MRI each year is also recommended.

After mastectomy, and even if the breast is reconstructed, a mammogram is not needed as there is negligible breast tissue to image, and any local recurrence should be detected as a nodule under the skin. However, if the nipple has been preserved sometimes an ultrasound of this area is suggested.

Regular blood tests or scans of the rest of the body have no real value in follow-up after early breast cancer as they are not likely to pick up recurrence before it presents with a symptom. However, if the patient has a persisting problem such as backache, headache, or lung issues, these should be discussed with the doctor and followed-up with scans and blood tests. Much research is going on to try to develop non-invasive tests such as a blood test that could detect recurrence early when intervention may improve the cure (circulating tumour cells and DNA are examples of these); however, to date these are not proven to be of benefit.

Side effects of treatment

An important role of follow-up is to monitor the patient for problems that may arise from the treatments used. This includes many of the issues discussed in Chapter 10, such as menopausal symptoms and bone health. It is important the patient discusses any problems with the oncologist or surgeon at the follow-up visit as most can be addressed and improved. A checklist of these is in the care plan detailed next.

As endocrine therapy must be taken for at least 5 and often 10 years, side effects during this time often come up between 6-monthly or annual visits. Taking a care plan to the GP to address these can be useful.

A care plan

This needs to include:

◆ A summary of the cancer diagnosis including dates, pathology details, and treating doctors

◆ A summary of treatments received including surgery (what, when, and by whom), radiotherapy, and drug treatments

◆ The oncologist's estimate of the chance of recurrence with treatment

◆ The recommended follow-up schedule including when to have a mammogram and ultrasound, and when visits to each specialist is due

◆ Potential late effects of each treatment including surgery, radiotherapy, chemo and hormone therapy, and anti-HER2 therapy

◆ What symptoms and side effects to report, for example, bone pain, shortness of breath, or headaches

◆ Identified concerns of the individual patient and where to refer these, which may include:

  ◆ Mood changes (psychology)

  ◆ Fertility (fertility specialist)

  ◆ Relationships (counsellor)

  ◆ Family history (genetic counsellor)

  ◆ Weight and exercise (exercise programme)

  ◆ Menopause (menopause clinic)

  ◆ Lymphedema (physiotherapist or occupational therapist)

  ◆ Osteoporosis (endocrinologist)

  ◆ Reconstruction (plastic surgeon)

Several care plans are featured at the end of this chapter, under 'Further resources'.

General practitioner follow-up

Increasingly cancer follow-up care is being shifted from what is seen as expensive, inefficient hospital care where a patient may see several different doctors with little coordination of care for the whole patient, to general practice. This can be a very good way to follow-up people after cancer as long as the GP has been adequately informed about the treatment the patient received and the nature of her cancer, and what problems to expect into the future. It is a very important to have a clear follow-up plan of when tests and check-ups are needed and for how long.

All patients who have had breast cancer need at least an annual physical examination along with a review of their medication and any potential side effects. Women who have not had bilateral mastectomy need an annual mammogram, and if they are on aromatase inhibitors they need a bone density scan every few years. It is important to have a rapid access pathway back to specialist care should any problems arise.

Ensuring the GP has a copy of a care plan will improve communication and ultimately care for the patient.

📄 Case study

Jill is a 49-year-old woman diagnosed a year ago with a small 10 mm ER-positive HER2-negative grade 1 cancer of the left breast, with one lymph node involved of twelve removed. She had undergone a hook-wire localized removal of the cancer and sentinel node biopsy followed by removal of more lymph nodes from under the arm. She then had 5 weeks of radiotherapy and tamoxifen, which she was still on.

Jill was otherwise pretty fit, weighing 60 kg and with a height of 165 cm, with a body mass index (BMI) of 22. She had recently joined a gym and was doing 30 minutes of moderate intensity aerobic exercise 4 days a week with some weights for resistance training and yoga on another day. As a vegetarian she had quite a low-fat diet but agreed to increase her intake of calcium, and a vitamin D blood test measure showed this to be low, so she started supplements. Jill enjoys drinking a few glasses of wine at the weekend and sometimes smokes a cigarette when drinking—she is trying to cut this out!

Jill was seen in a special 'Healthy Living after Breast Cancer clinic' by a doctor and a follow-up and care plan devised for her. This included the need for 6-monthly follow-up by her oncologist and surgeon alternating until

5 years, then every year for another 5 years, and annual mammogram and ultrasound of the breasts for life. She was also taught how to examine her breasts and was informed about being aware of any new changes in them.

Since starting tamoxifen she has noted some hot flushes and her periods have stopped. However, these flushes are mild and she is happy just to monitor these and wear clothing in layers if she needs to strip some off when hot.

One of her main issues is stiffness in the arm of her left side and some swelling and discomfort in the left breast. She has only seen a physiotherapist once before surgery so agreed to go back to a physio to see if this can be helped, and was recommended a compression bra to ease the mild lymphoedema in the breast.

Jill was asked how much she worried about cancer recurrence. Although she was obviously concerned about this, the thoughts were not unduly intrusive and she had good support networks and good communication with both her family and friends which she felt made her recovery easier. She was more concerned about the effects on the radiation on her heart and lungs and agreed that giving up smoking was a good plan to improve her health in this regard. She was also urged to establish a good relationship with a regular GP—something she had never had—to address preventative health issue and for peace of mind.

Further resources

Care plans

Cancer.Net. *ASCO Cancer Treatment and Survivorship Care Plans*. Available at: http://www.cancer.net/survivorship/follow-care-after-cancer-treatment/asco-cancer-treatment-and-survivorship-care-plans

Government of Western Australia, Department of Health. *Breast Cancer Survivorship Care Plan*. Available at: http://www.healthnetworks.health.wa.gov.au/cancer/docs/Breast%20collaborative%20survivorship%20care%20plan%20-%20personnalised%20version.pdf

Journey Forward. *Cancer Survivorship Care Plan*. Available at: https://www.journeyforward.org/sites/journeyforward/files/sample-care-plan_breast-cancer.pdf

12

Advanced (metastatic) and recurrent cancer

 Key points

♦ Local recurrence is when breast cancer returns and involves regional lymph nodes or chest wall, or in distant sites in the body

♦ Metastatic cancer or distant recurrence is when disease has spread to other areas of the body. Drug therapies are usually the main modality in this setting

♦ Clinical trials of new drugs should be considered for patients with metastatic breast cancer

Advanced breast cancer can mean two different things, either locally advanced (see Chapter 9) or metastatic. Patients diagnosed with locally advanced or metastatic cancer have quite different treatment pathways.

Recurrent and metastatic breast cancer

Recurrent breast cancer means cancer that has returned after the first diagnosis of breast cancer, and is the same tumour as the first cancer. This is in contrast to a 'second primary', or new breast cancer, which can occur in the same or other breast. Recurrence can be local and thus occur in the conserved breast or in the skin and soft tissues over the chest wall after mastectomy, or occasionally in lymph nodes under the arm. It can also be at a distant site in the body, such as the bone or an organ, so is called metastatic cancer. Even if the recurrence is apparently just local, it is important to have scans to check it has not spread elsewhere too.

Local recurrences are usually treated with local therapies, surgery if possible, which may mean a completion mastectomy or axillary clearance or removing a nodule from the skin. If radiotherapy has not been given this can be a good treatment. Very occasionally it can be give twice to small areas. Systemic therapies are also used in this setting, particularly if the local recurrence is not amenable to local therapies or if the local recurrence occurs after previous surgery and radiotherapy.

Distant recurrences are when the cancer recurs in other parts of the body, otherwise known as metastatic disease. Metastatic breast cancer is not curable in most cases. The prognosis depends on several factors, and features associated with better outcomes include a longer duration between the first cancer and the recurrence, hormone receptor-positive disease, metastasis to the bone only, and if the person is generally fitter.

Metastases from breast cancer are most commonly found in bones, but can also be to the lungs, liver, brain, and less often to other sites. These areas of cancer can be silent without symptoms. General symptoms include fatigue, weight loss, and loss of appetite. Other symptoms tend to be specific to the site of metastases. Bone metastases can cause aches and pains in the bones, low blood counts as the bone marrow is where these cells are produced, or high circulating calcium levels as a result of the affected bone releasing calcium into the blood stream. Lung metastases can result in shortness of breath or a cough. Liver metastases, if very large, can cause abdominal pain or jaundice (yellowing of the eyes and skin). Brain metastases can cause confusion or other mental changes. It is important to note that metastases occur in a minority of patients with breast cancer, and these symptoms are much more likely to be due to a variety of unrelated benign conditions (see Table 12.1).

Occasionally at first diagnosis of breast cancer the disease has already spread, so is metastatic (also known as Stage 4 cancer). This is only seen in around 2 in every 100 patients presenting with breast cancer and is usually found on tests done because the patient has a very aggressive local cancer in the breast. Sometimes the actual metastasis is the first symptom that presents, without a lump in the breast.

Table 12.1 Symptoms of breast cancer spread or metastasis

Site	Symptom
Local recurrence	Nodule often near scar
Bone	Pain, fracture, or anaemia
Liver	Abdominal pain and bloating or jaundice
Lungs	Cough or shortness of breath
Brain	Headaches or faints

This can cause difficulties in diagnosis as it may be hard to biopsy a metastasis in some organs, and the actual breast cancer in the breast can be very small.

Although not curable in the majority of cases, most patients with metastatic breast cancer are able to continue normal lives for many years after diagnosis with appropriate treatment. Treatment of metastatic breast cancer depends on the site of metastasis, the subtype of tumour, the symptoms experienced by the patient, prior therapies received, and the general well-being of the patient. A biopsy of the metastasis may be done to see if the pathology of the tumour has changed over time, which will dictate the new treatment recommended. Molecular tests are also sometimes used at this point on the biopsy of the metastasis, as a tool to look for novel therapeutic targets in the cancer. This may be done in the context of a research study, although there are commercial companies such as Foundation One that offer this test.

The primary mode of treatment in metastatic breast cancer is systemic or drug therapies, as such an approach will target multiple sites of metastatic disease, as opposed to surgery and radiotherapy, which typically only focus on one or two sites of disease. These treatments are rarely curative and are aimed at prolonging the duration and quality of life. The drug therapies used are similar to those used for early stage breast cancer, as described in Chapter 8. If the patient has not received prior drug treatment for breast cancer, it would be likely that one of the treatments used for early stage breast cancer is used as the patient's cancer is considered treatment naïve and so still potentially sensitive to this drug. There are additional drugs that have been shown to be effective in metastatic and treatment-resistant settings to the therapies listed in Chapter 8, and clinical trials of new drugs are usually first evaluated in patients with metastatic disease. It is critical that the side effect profile and the patient's fitness for treatment be carefully considered, as the primary goals of therapy are not only to increase duration of life, but also improve quality of life. It is important that the patient is not made miserable with drug side effects if their lifespan is limited, and as the treatment not curative.

The role of local therapies in metastatic disease is very limited. Radiotherapy is very useful for painful bone metastases (usually a short 5-day course) and can also be used to treat some liver and brain lesions. Surgery can sometimes be used to remove single sites of disease, such as in the brain or liver.

Endocrine therapies and combinations for metastatic breast cancer

While tamoxifen, aromatase inhibitors, and gonadotrophin-releasing hormone (GnRH) analogues are effective in treating hormone receptor-positive early breast cancer, a proportion of patients will relapse from their disease. These cancers may be inherently resistant or develop resistance to endocrine therapies. There are many mechanisms of resistance to endocrine therapies, including mutations that arise in the oestrogen receptor (ER) gene that result in the receptor being perpetually being turned on, thereby rendering conventional therapies ineffective. Another mechanism of endocrine resistance is the switching on of alternative growth pathways. Typically, when endocrine therapies stop working, the only options left for the patient are chemotherapy and clinical trials of experimental treatments. There have been several developments aimed at extending the use of endocrine therapies, either with newer classes of endocrine therapies, such as selective oestrogen receptor degraders (SERDs) such as fulvestrant (Faslodex), or by combining endocrine therapies with drugs that target the alternate growth pathways that are switched on in endocrine-resistant breast cancer. Two such types of drugs that have been shown to be effective include mTOR inhibitors and cyclin-dependent kinase 4 and 6 inhibitors. These are described below.

Fulvestrant (Faslodex)

Fulvestrant belongs to a class of drugs called SERDs, which act by breaking down the ER in cancer cells, and thereby inhibiting its growth promoting properties. This drug has been shown to be effective in patients whose cancers have progressed on prior treatment with tamoxifen and aromatase inhibitors. It has also shown to be effective in patients who have not previously received other forms of endocrine therapy. It is given as a monthly injection. Next-generation SERDs are currently being developed that are more potent and administered orally.

Everolimus (Afinitor)

Everolimus is a targeted therapy that inhibits a protein called mammalian target of rapamycin (mTOR), which is a key molecule in an alternative cancer growth pathway that is switched on in endocrine-resistant breast cancer. It is also approved for use in several other cancer types. It is licensed for use in combination with endocrine therapies in endocrine-resistant recurrent breast cancer. Everolimus comes in the form of a tablet, and its common side effects include fatigue and mouth ulcers. Rarely, patients can develop inflammation of their lungs.

Cyclin-dependent kinase 4 and 6 (CDK4/6) inhibitors

CDK4/6 inhibitors have recently been approved in many countries for use in combination with endocrine therapy for endocrine-resistant metastatic breast cancer. This combination currently represents the most effective therapy in the first-line treatment of ER-positive, HER2-negative metastatic breast cancer. There are several drugs in this class, including palbociclib (Ibrance), ribociclib (Kisqali), and abemaciclib (Verzenio). This class of drugs comes in the form of tablets, and is associated with the side effects of low blood count, fatigue, and diarrhoea. Trials are underway to evaluate the efficacy of this class of drug in ER-positive, HER2-positive breast cancer.

HER2-directed therapies
for metastatic disease

While trastuzumab and pertuzumab and chemotherapy combinations are effective in treating HER2-positive early stage breast cancer, a proportion of patients will relapse from their disease. These cancers may be inherently resistant or develop resistance to these therapies. In women with metastatic breast cancer, trastuzumab can be combined with several chemotherapy agents, or given alone. Pertuzumab is effective in combination with trastuzumab and chemotherapy for the treatment of metastatic HER2-positive breast cancer, and this combination of both anti-HER2 drugs with chemotherapy currently represents the most effective first-line therapy in women with metastatic HER2-positive breast cancer.

Trastuzumab emtansine (T-DM1, or
Kadcyla)

T-DM1 is a type of HER2-directed therapy comprising trastuzumab linked to a small amount of chemotherapy called emtansine. This antibody-chemotherapy conjugate acts by combining the specificity of the HER2 antibody and the anticancer effects of chemotherapy. The chemotherapy is directed only to the cancer cells and not the rest of the body, making it effective with less side effects. This is given intravenously every 3 weeks, and in addition to the side effects of trastuzumab, can also result in low platelet counts and a degree of liver inflammation. In general, it is better tolerated than normal chemotherapy. T-DM1 is currently only licensed for use in patients with metastatic breast cancer. However, it is being clinically evaluated in early stage breast cancer.

Lapatinib (Tykerb)

Lapatinib is another class of HER2-directed therapies. Unlike the previous anti-HER2 drugs, lapatinib is not an antibody but an inhibitor of an enzyme, tyrosine kinase. It is administered as a tablet orally, and used in combination with chemotherapy. It is only approved for use in the setting of metastatic breast cancer. Side effects are not uncommon with lapatinib-based combination treatments, which include diarrhoea and fatigue.

Chemotherapy for metastatic disease

There are a few key differences between chemotherapy use in metastatic and early stage breast cancer. However, there are more chemotherapy options that are used in metastatic breast cancer than early stage breast cancer. Chemotherapy is also more often used as a single agent one after another (sequential treatment) over some months or years in patients with metastatic breast cancer, in contrast to combination therapy of two or three drugs together in early stage breast cancer. The reason for this is that as the disease is not curable, a sequential single treatment approach allows for spacing out of the therapies, and importantly, maintaining a better quality of life. It also allows for the potential of a longer treatment duration as opposed to chemotherapy for early stage breast cancer, which is more taxing on the body and is typically limited to a few months' duration.

Chemotherapies used in metastatic breast cancer include anthracyclines such as doxorubicin (adriamycin), epirubicin, and liposomal doxorubicin (caelyx); microtubule inhibitors including taxanes such as paclitaxel (taxol), nab-paclitaxel (abraxane), and docetaxel (taxotere), vinorelbine (navelbine), and eribulin (havalen); antimetabolites such as capecitabine (xeloda), gemcitabine (gemzar), and methotrexate; and platinums such as cisplatin and carboplatin.

Other systemic therapies for metastatic disease

Bone-directed therapies

For patients with metastasis to the bone or with high levels of circulating calcium, bone-directed therapies have been shown to reduce fracture rates and normalize calcium levels. Therapies include bisphosphonates, such as zoledronic acid (Zometa), aledronate, clodronate, and pamidronate; as well Denosumab (Xgeva), an antibody that works by preventing the development of osteoclasts, which are cells that break down bone.

Poly ADP ribose polymerase (PARP) inhibitors

A new class of drugs called PARP inhibitors have recently been shown to specifically target cancer cells that have lost their ability to repair their faulty genes

(DNA). These tumours are the type found in women who carry an inherited gene fault in the *BRCA1* and *BRCA2* genes (see Chapter 2). PARP inhibitors selectively kill cells where this form of DNA repair is absent, and so are highly effective in killing tumour cells with a mutated form of *BRCA* gene. Normal cells are largely unaffected by the drug as they still possess this crucial DNA repair mechanism. These drugs have been approved for use in patients with metastatic ovarian cancer and breast cancer in the setting of *BRCA* gene mutations.

Clinical trials

Most advances in medicine have come from the laboratory and from experiments in cell cultures or mice; however, it is vitally important these advances are tested in humans with the disease. Thus, clinical trials are the type of research performed in patients that can tell us the tolerability of new therapies, that is, if they have acceptable side effects, and if one treatment is better than another. Clinical trials are carefully worked out studies, which must be approved by the ethics and scientific committees at each hospital where they are being run. These are typically conducted at tertiary specialist referral centres.

Participating in a clinical trial is an altruistic act that may not be of any specific advantage to the individual. However, many patients with breast cancer feel it is important to do so, as they will be helping the next generation of patients with the disease. It also means a patient may receive a new treatment that is currently not approved for routine use in breast cancer, thereby representing an added treatment option. The close monitoring and follow-up patients receive in clinical trials, along with the fact that they are usually conducted by centres with a specific interest in the disease, means patients in trials tend to have better outcomes than those not in them.

Coping with recurrent and metastatic disease

Being diagnosed with recurrent breast cancer can be more devastating even than the original diagnosis. Knowing the disease has spread and so may not be curable is frightening and challenging.

People with advanced cancer are more likely to develop depression and other psychological issues, as well as potentially coping with physical symptoms such as discomfort or pain, fatigue, and treatment side effects.

Ensuring a good diet and, if possible, an exercise programme will help with both symptoms and quality of life—many exercise programmes are now available targeted at people with advanced cancer. Addressing practical issues is also important—getting help around the house, getting financial advice, considering accessing pension plans or superannuation, and legal advice about a will.

However, many people will benefit from specialist psychology support at this time which can be accessed through both specialist doctors and breast nurses, or through many charitable organizations.

Palliative and supportive care

Therapies that focus on symptom management are very important in the management of metastatic breast cancer. These include treatments to alleviate pain (from simple analgesics to more potent ones such as opioids), nausea, and depression. This is sometimes done in consultation with palliative care physicians who specialize in these treatments. Palliative care means controlling symptoms in association with optimizing emotional, social, and spiritual well-being. Many people fear the idea of palliative care as they feel it is 'giving up treatment'. In fact, it is far from this and may involve many active treatments or be offered at the same time as active cancer treatments are given. It is aimed to give the person the best quality of life when they are unlikely to be cured from their cancer.

Palliative care is practised by both specialist palliative care physicians and specialist nurses and can be delivered in hospital, at home, or in a hospice. Most oncologists work closely with palliative care colleagues, as do GPs who are often trained in this area as well. Palliative care addresses the symptoms which a person with advanced cancer may experience such as pain, breathlessness, or nausea, can deal with wound problems, and plan for any future care crisis. They will also provide support to both the patient and carers, and offer help during bereavement. Planning for the end of life with dignity and without pain or other debilitating symptoms is a vital part of coping with advanced breast cancer. Increasingly, palliative care support is being offered to patients at home in addition to a hospice, giving patients another option for their end of life care.

Some patients use complementary treatments when diagnosed with advanced disease. These can be very helpful in alleviating symptoms and are discussed in Chapter 10. It is critical that these treatments be discussed with the treating team as they may affect the efficacy of the anticancer treatments through drug interactions.

📄 Case study

Olivia is a 61-year-old woman who was first diagnosed with breast cancer in her right breast 5 years before, when she had noted a lump. She went on to have surgery including a mastectomy and axillary clearance for what was a 3 cm ER-positive, PR-negative, HER2-negative cancer, which was also in four lymph nodes. She had chemotherapy and radiotherapy and is on an aromatase inhibitor drug.

For the last few months Olivia has been experiencing lower back pain which she initially attributed to moving some furniture, but when it did not improve with time and painkillers, she attended her GP. He quickly referred her back to her oncologist who ordered several scans and blood tests. These show that Olivia now has cancer back in her bones—in her lower spine and left hip. She had a short course of radiotherapy to her spine to help with the pain, and was started on a combination of the endocrine therapy along with palbociclib, which belongs to a new class of drug called CDK4/6 inhibitors. The oncologist has also recommended the bone-modifying drug denosumab, and in the short term, some stronger painkillers.

Olivia was devastated to hear the cancer had returned—she felt almost worse than at first diagnosis. However, she is relieved to hear the disease seems to be just in the bone and hopefully the drugs can control the disease and her symptoms for many, many years.

Further resources

Breast Cancer Network Australia. *Metastatic Breast Cancer*. Available at: https://www.bcna.org.au/metastatic-breast-cancer/

Breast Cancer Research Foundation. *The Progress Report*. Available at: https://www.bcrf.org/blog/asco-2017-updates-clinical-trialspalliativecare.org.au

Cancer Australia. *Locally Advanced Breast Cancer*. Available at: https://breast-cancer.canceraustralia.gov.au/types/locally-advanced-breast-cancer

NIH National Cancer Institute. *Metastatic Cancer*. Available at: https://www.cancer.gov/types/metastatic-cancer

Susan G. Komen. *Metastatic Breast Cancer*. Available at: https://ww5.komen.org/BreastCancer/MetastaticBreastCancerIntroduction.html

13

For the partners, family, friends, and colleagues affected by breast cancer

 Key points

- Getting informed about breast cancer and its treatment will help you support the person with the disease

- It is important to discuss how YOU feel, and not become isolated or distressed

- Make time to spend with the person with breast cancer—and work on the communication

- Inform children with age-appropriate language

More than one and a half million people each year are diagnosed with breast cancer worldwide, but many millions more will be affected by it—as partners, children, other family members, friends, and colleagues of those diagnosed. This chapter explores how you can effectively support someone close to you with breast cancer and how you can inform yourself about the disease and treatments they may be undergoing.

Being a partner of someone with breast cancer

Partners naturally are worried about their loved one's diagnosis with a potentially life-threatening disease but often feel frustrated that the situation is not in their control, and they may be worried about how they will cope with changes in the person with cancer—both physical and emotional. Often a partner will feel isolated with no one to discuss their feelings with, as they are reluctant to burden the person with cancer who is going through treatment.

These feeling are normal. Getting information about cancer and treatments can help, as can getting organized, being practical, and asking for help from others if needed. Making time to spend with each other, even having fun, can both maintain and improve a relationship. Communication is always important. If you continue to struggle, advice from a psychologist can be useful.

Children

Most children will realize there is something wrong even without being told, so talking to children about the cancer and treatments will help them cope. Some children develop behavioural issues—if very young they may become 'clingy', and older children may not want to go to school or can become anxious and withdrawn. Information, open communication, and allowing everyone to have a job to do and prove useful often helps. It is okay to talk about cancer and some find a support group useful. At the end of this chapter are some really good resources to help both children and their friends, teachers, and other adults.

Cultural differences and breast cancer

For people from some cultures breast cancer is more difficult to discuss, particularly with friends and colleagues. This is not just because of language barriers, but it may be because of embarrassment that a person has cancer, or that the cancer is in a private part of the body or that it somehow affects the person's 'womanhood'. Cultural experiences of medical treatment and fear of treatment and death also can be important issues.

Cultural and personal sensitivity in discussing a person's cancer and treatment are always important. But just showing you care with a kind word and perhaps some practical help is always welcome. People with cancer often report that some friends and acquaintances shun them after a cancer diagnosis—this is probably just fear of not saying or doing the correct thing. So make sure the person with cancer feels you are there to support them.

Breast cancer and work

For women who continue to work through their breast cancer treatment, telling their employer can be difficult. However, it is important to be open about treatment in order to plan work around it and any problems that may arise needing time off. This does not mean a person with breast cancer has to tell her entire workplace—her privacy is important. However, the human resources (HR) department (if there is one) will need some details.

It is also important to be realistic in what work can and cannot be done when undergoing treatments, so things are fair both for the person with cancer but also their colleagues and employer who may need to cover for them.

If time off is required, a plan to come back to work in stages may be useful, and good communication usually results in a supportive employer.

Many women value not only the continued financial benefits of working but also the normality of going to work. Work colleagues can thus support a person with breast cancer by good communication—listening and caring—and help make life easier in small practical ways.

How to support a woman with breast cancer

Ask her how she feels—communicate

Practical help—looking after the children, doing some house or garden work, driving her to appointments

Spoil her a little—arrange a massage or special treat (but remember she may feel tired and unwell and not want to be very active)

 Case study

Nigel's wife Glenys was recently diagnosed with a locally advanced breast cancer called an inflammatory cancer. She was undergoing chemotherapy and will then need to have a mastectomy and radiotherapy. Glenys seemed to be coping quite well with treatment and had a good network of friends and a close relationship with her grown-up daughter.

Nigel had found it difficult to talk to Glenys about the cancer. His own mother had died when he was quite young from breast cancer and he found himself obsessing about those memories and too worried to talk to Glenys about this. He found visits to the hospital particularly traumatic but felt he had to go with his wife to support her.

Their daughter could see the difficulty her dad was having so called a family meeting to discuss the cancer and how they were going to tackle it. Even being able to all talk for a few hours felt better for Nigel. And at a subsequent visit to the hospital they brought this up with the oncologist and breast nurse who were able to reassure them that this was normal, and that with some counselling both Nigel and Glenys could develop better communication.

Nigel realized that he was a great support for his wife—and that just being there made her feel better. He was able to discuss some of his fears with a counsellor and gradually began to overcome them. Glenys did very well through treatment and they planned a long-awaited cruise at the end of it, which gave then not only something to look forward to but valuable time together also.

Looking back, Nigel said that although Glenys's cancer was one of the worst times of their lives, it had made the family stronger.

Further resources

Breast Cancer Network Australia. *Information for Partners*. Available at: https://www.bcna.org.au/understanding-breast-cancer/talking-to-family-and-friends/information-for-partners/

Cancer Australia. *Managing Emotional Changes Due to Breast Cancer*. Available at: https://canceraustralia.gov.au/affected-cancer/cancer-types/breast-cancer/living-breast-cancer/managing-emotional-changes-due-breast-cancer/impact-breast-cancer-diagnosis-partners

Facing Cancer Together. *Caregivers and Family Resources*. Available at: https://facingcancertogether.witf.org/resources/caregivers-family-resources-33111

The Gathering Place. *Explaining Cancer to Kids*. Available at: http://www.someoneiloveissick.com/talking-to-your-children-about-cancer/explaining-cancer-to-kids/

Very Well Health. *Breast Cancer Work Rights and Legal Provisions*. Available at: https://www.verywell.com/breast-cancer-and-work-your-rights-and-legal-provisions-430702

14

Special situations

 Key points

◆ Breast cancer diagnosed during pregnancy has similar outcomes of that in other young women

◆ Surgery and chemotherapy can be given during pregnancy

◆ Around 6% of breast cancer occurs in women under 40

◆ Breast cancer in young women is more likely to be associated with an inherited gene fault

◆ If elderly but fit, surgery is suitable for most patients

Pregnancy and breast cancer

Breast cancer is fortunately a very rare event in pregnant and breastfeeding women, but does occur in about 5% of women under 45 who are diagnosed with cancer when either pregnant or breastfeeding. Any woman who has a persistent breast symptom at any age, and even if pregnant, needs to have it thoroughly checked out. Even during pregnancy, a woman can have breast imaging with an ultrasound, and often a mammogram can be performed with shielding of the baby from the X-rays. Needle tests are also possible although the pathologist needs to be made aware of the pregnancy in order to properly assess the specimen. During breastfeeding it can be more difficult to do a biopsy as milk can leak through the biopsy tract.

If cancer is diagnosed it is important that the woman is looked after by a specialist team, preferably ones experienced in this area, as both the mother and baby require expert care. Breast cancer is always a devastating diagnosis but most women can be very effectively treated and the outcomes for women diagnosed during pregnancy are similar to women diagnosed while not pregnant. Unless a woman is in the very early stages of pregnancy and needs chemotherapy, there is no reason to consider termination of the pregnancy unless this is her wish.

Surgery can be performed during pregnancy, but is more likely to be a mast-ectomy as the cancers can be quite large and breast-conserving surgery more difficult in a pregnant breast. It is best to consider a delayed reconstruction. Radiotherapy cannot be given during pregnancy due to the dangers to the un-born child, so needs to wait until after delivery.

Chemotherapy can be safely given during pregnancy after the first trimester (week 12) although the drug Herceptin is not recommended, nor are hormonal drugs such as tamoxifen as they can all affect the baby. It is important to time delivery of the baby carefully to allow any effects of chemotherapy to wear off. Many women will undergo slightly early delivery at about 38 weeks, which is quite safe for the baby, and although the caesarean section rate is higher, normal vaginal delivery is certainly possible for many women. Breastfeeding afterwards is only possible if the patient is not on any chemotherapy drugs—sometimes stopping these for a few weeks to allow at least a brief period of breastfeeding is possible.

Sometimes breast cancer is detected during breastfeeding or just after when the breasts stop producing milk and become much easier to feel.

Young women with breast cancer

Breast cancer is uncommon in young women but nevertheless around 1 in 2,000 women in their twenties will develop the disease and 1 in 300 in their thirties. Around 6% of breast cancers occur in this age group. Because these women are not having screening mammograms most will find a lump them-selves and often the cancer is somewhat larger than in older women. If a symptom such as a lump is found it should be investigated by a doctor with a clinical breast examination and, if needed, an ultrasound and needle biopsy. Most lumps will be benign, for example, cysts or a fibroadenoma (a harmless lump which is thought to be due to a lobule in the breast enlarging into a lump, but which does need to be confirmed as such with a needle biopsy). However, if the symptom is suspicious a mammogram can be useful.

Cancers in very young women are more likely to be related to an inherited gene fault and so these women may have a strong family history of breast and/or ovarian cancer or other cancers. It is appropriate to refer most women under 40 with breast cancer to a familial cancer service to consider genetic testing. However, 80% will not have a gene fault found although a strong family history even without a gene fault does mean the family should discuss this risk with a genetic expert.

Cancers in young women also tend to be more aggressive with more oestrogen-receptor (ER)- and progesterone-receptor (PR)-negative, grade 3 cancers, and so a somewhat worse outlook—overall around 90% of women with breast cancer can expect to be alive and cancer-free after diagnosis. This is nearer 85% for younger women.

Young women with breast cancer often do face a particular set of problems. These include issues around relationships and children, more psychological stress, body image issues, and work and financial pressures.

Relationship issues may be that the woman is not in one! And starting a relationship after cancer treatment can be hard—especially dealing with some of the physical issues such as having a mastectomy. If the woman is in a relationship it may be early on in it, or a casual one, and her partner and she will face challenges maintaining the relationship. If she does not have children or wishes to have more, she may need to consider this casual partner to be the one with whom to make embryos before starting chemotherapy.

Coping with young children can also be hard while undergoing cancer treatment. Both practical and emotional issues loom large, and the breast cancer nurse is well placed to advise on many of these, as well as access practical help and childcare. Asking for help from other school mums and friends often brings in lots offers of help and support—it is worth asking! Issues around future fertility are discussed in Chapter 10.

Loss of income, loss of pension, and difficulties in obtaining insurance or a mortgage are real problems facing some young women with breast cancer. This may be made worse if the patient has to pay for some of her treatment. Some local cancer organizations or the social work department of the hospital can help address these issues. If a woman does need to take significant time off work (which most do), discussing the reason for this with the employer should lead them to be supportive. Contacting a union representative can also help.

Breast cancer in older and frail people

Older women who develop breast cancer face many challenges, which may largely be due to having several coexisting medical conditions, but also because they may not have much support and find some treatments harder to tolerate.

If a patient is fit enough to tolerate an anaesthetic, surgery is the best first-line treatment for a breast cancer to allow good local control, and may mean the patient does not need any further treatments. Mastectomy is usually very well tolerated by older women and may mean they do not require radiotherapy which is often hard to get to every day.

If the patient is not fit for surgery and the cancer is ER positive, treatment with tamoxifen or an aromatase inhibitor tablet is usually very effective at least for some years, with minimal side effects. Close monitoring every 4–6 months is usually arranged.

Chemotherapy is harder to tolerate and not so effective in older women. However, how old is 'old' is dependent not so much on chronological age but on fitness—and certainly some women in their eighties can manage more gentle weekly intravenous or oral chemotherapy very well.

The important balance is to keep an older person as fit and symptom-free as long as possible, and not let the cancer or treatment impact too much on their quality of life.

The 'Further resources' section at the end of this chapter lists several websites to help answer the many questions a patient or her family may have about breast cancer in older people.

Phyllodes tumours

This relatively rare group of tumours range from benign lumps, very much like a fibroadenoma but which can grow quite quickly and need surgical removal, to extremely rarely malignant tumours that can spread and prove fatal.

Any fast-growing lump needs investigation and probably surgical removal. If the lump turns out on pathology testing to be a phyllodes tumour, most will be benign with no further treatment needed as long as the lump is completely removed. However, some are 'borderline' tumours which need careful follow-up with ultrasound, and very rarely will be malignant which will then need referral to an oncologist and sometimes chemotherapy.

📄 Case study

Tanya, a 29-year-old administration assistant, had just finished breast-feeding her first child, now 6 months old, when she realized the knotty lump in her left breast was not getting smaller, even though her breasts were going back to their prepregnant state. Her paternal grandmother had developed breast cancer in her thirties so Tanya was understandably worried about this lump, even though she had been reassured during breastfeeding the lumpy area was normal. Investigations by her GP revealed a 2 cm breast cancer of a 'triple negative' type. She was advised to undergo chemotherapy followed by surgery.

Tanya and her partner had planned to have a second child and she was really keen to keep this as an option. She and Steve, her partner, were referred to a fertility specialist and she underwent a cycle of *in vitro* fertilization (IVF) before chemotherapy started and three embryos were stored.

During chemotherapy Tanya saw a family cancer clinic. After counselling, she underwent genetic testing which revealed an inherited gene fault in the *BRCA1* gene. After 6 months of chemotherapy she opted to have a bilateral mastectomy and immediate reconstruction with implants, as she knew the gene fault put her at higher risk of a second breast cancer in the future.

Two years on Tanya was well and pretty much completely recovered from the cancer journey. She decided to attempt another pregnancy and underwent preimplantation genetic testing of her stored embryos—so one was implanted which did not carry the *BRCA* gene. Nine months later Tanya and Steve had a second baby daughter—and completed their family.

Further resources

Breast Cancer WA. *Young Women and Breast Cancer*. Available at: http://www.breastcancer.org.au/about-breast-cancer/young-women-and-breast-cancer.aspx

Breastcancer.org. *Symptoms and Diagnosis of Phyllodes Tumors of the Breast*. Available at: http://www.breastcancer.org/symptoms/types/phyllodes/diagnosis

Cancer Care. *Questions and Answers about Elderly*. Available at: http://www.cancercare.org/questions/tagged/elderly

Susan G. Komen. *Unique Issues for Young Women with Breast Cancer*. Available at: http://ww5.komen.org/BreastCancer/YoungWomenandBreastCancer.html

15

The future—what tests and treatments may be around the corner

 Key points

- Drugs to prevent breast cancer in women at higher risk
- A liquid biopsy may be able to detect tiny fragments of tumour DNA in blood
- Breast reconstruction techniques may include growing a new breast from fat stem cells
- Molecular tests may establish who can avoid radiotherapy
- Drugs targeted at aberrant tumour pathways will improve survival
- The patient's own immune system may be re-programmed to fight the cancer

Huge advances have been made in the detection and treatment of breast cancer over the last 30 years. Survival has increased from 70% of women surviving the diagnosis of breast cancer 25 years ago to more than 90% in most Western countries. And for most women, although treatment will still be somewhat arduous and side effects and complications certainly will affect many, lots of support is available to help them get through it and most will make a complete recovery and return to a 'new normal' life.

These improvements in length and quality of life have come about due to research into better ways of diagnosing and treating people with breast cancer, and research continues to be the key to further improvements in outcomes.

However, more than a million and a half women each year will still be diagnosed with breast cancer—so we need to lower the numbers of women who develop the disease (incidence)—and thus prevent cancer developing. Of those who do develop breast cancer, too many will still suffer a recurrence of their cancer and even die of the disease—until this is zero, more research is needed into better treatments. And we need to find treatments that will not only be tailored to the individual and her cancer, but will cause only minimal side effects, be easy to tolerate, and allow women to return to a fully functional life without long-term side effects.

Clinical trials

The way we try to understand if a potential new treatment is better than current ones is by doing a study called a clinical trial. A trial will also need to find out what side effects the new treatment may have and how safe it is. Many trials are randomized so the trial participant will have either the current 'usual' treatment or a new one, and the process for choosing this is done randomly by a computer. This is to avoid bias, which means the human element of the doctor or researcher, even unconsciously, trying to choose which treatment may be better for an individual. This bias would mean we could never truly know if the new treatment is better.

Clinical trials can be done for new drug treatments but also for other treatments, such as whether a certain exercise programme improves how a patient feels after cancer, or for new tests such as a new laboratory test to better categorize what kind of cancer it is under the microscope.

Preventing breast cancer

Advances have come in preventing breast cancer mainly by looking at existing drugs—we now know that antihormone drugs such as tamoxifen and the aromatase inhibitors halve the chance of developing oestrogen-receptor (ER) positive breast cancer in women at risk of this. In many countries these are now available to be prescribed. However, these drugs have not been shown to decrease the overall chance of dying from breast cancer and do have considerable side effects for some women. This means they are unlikely to be used by large numbers of women.

One key to improving this is to find a way of accurately assessing an individual's risk of developing breast cancer and then developing individualized strategies to help her minimize this risk. Current research has developed computer modelling solutions which are able to be used, for example, in the general practitioner's surgery to assess an individual's risk using information such as her family history, her body mass index (BMI), and mammographic density, and a blood test looking at some genetic risk factors, and then develop a plan to minimize her risk. This plan may include an exercise and weight loss programme, a plan of how often she needs surveillance imaging and what this should be (such as just mammograms or MRI), and if she should consider risk-reducing drugs. One such programme can be found at https://www.petermac.org\iprevent.

Other new research is looking at using a drug normally used to treat osteoporosis and bone metastases called denosumab to lower the risk of breast cancer in women carrying the *BRCA* gene. If successful, this may not get rid of risk completely in these women but will, we hope, allow them some years before making decisions on prophylactic surgery.

We are beginning to realize the vital importance of a healthy lifestyle in preventing some cancers and in preventing recurrence in women who have had cancer. Recent research has now established how much exercise is needed (at least 150 minutes each week of exercise which makes you sweaty and breathless) and 'wearable technologies' (similar to the Fitbit) are being developed to help people track and maintain their health.

Detecting breast cancer

New screening and imaging tests for breast cancer include molecular imaging techniques that use radioactive tracers that light up areas of cancer within the breast. One of these already showing promise is scintimammography, which uses a radioactive tracer injected into the vein and a special camera which detects if the tracer attaches to cancer cells in the breast. Its routine place is still not clear, but it may prove better than conventional mammography in younger women with dense breasts. Newer mammography and ultrasound techniques using contrast agents and sophisticated computing are also improving detection rates for cancers. MRI is getting faster and cheaper (ultra-fast MRI) and may well be offered to many more women in the near future.

One very exciting area of detection research is using an engineering technique called micro-elastography to look for microscopic residual cells in the breast after the cancer has been removed, allowing the woman and her surgeon to be sure all cancer is gone and the all-too-common scenario of a second operation to remove 'margins' is not needed (https://www.oncoresmedical.com/). While still in the development phase, this technology, and others like it, may make surgery much easier in the future.

Other ways to detect cancer early and monitor its progress and response to treatment are the subject of much current research. We can already measure

121

from a simple blood test circulating tumour cells and fragments of tumour which we know correlate with prognosis and treatment response. These are not yet ready to use in the clinic for patients but may very soon be. The hope is that a simple blood test (a 'liquid biopsy') looking either for circulating tumour cells or for tiny fragments of tumour DNA in the blood stream could either detect cancer very early or detect if it is spreading. Further exciting work is then going on to try to stop this cancer spread—such as some very novel small implantable scaffold devices soaked in immune cells, designed to capture cancer cells as they begin to travel through the body.

Surgical advances

While more than half of women with breast cancer no longer need a mastectomy, and increasing numbers do not need all their lymph nodes removed from under the arm, there is still a long way to go to improve surgery and the outcomes from it for patients.

Research is even trying to establish if some women need no surgery at all—for example, those with very low-risk cancer such as some ductal carcinoma *in situ* (DCIS) (being studied in the US COMET trial and in the UK LORIS trial). Also being trialled is 'minimally invasive' surgery, using lasers, for example, for very small good outlook tumours. For those who respond very well to upfront drug treatment (neoadjuvant chemotherapy), where the tumour in the breast and lymph nodes seems to disappear completely on imaging tests, the hope is that in the future they also will be able to avoid surgery.

Oncoplastic breast surgery is now commonplace (see Chapter 6) and if a woman does need a mastectomy, in most cases she can be offered reconstruction. Techniques for this are rapidly changing—new materials to cover implants are being used—some made from human or animal material and some from synthetic material. These allow more women to have implant reconstruction and we hope will improve the appearance of these reconstructions.

Plastic surgeons are also pioneering new types of reconstruction such as the profunda artery perforator (PAP) flap where the fat along the buttock crease is used to reconstruct a breast.

Lipomodelling, where fat is sucked out of the tummy or thigh and injected over a reconstruction or to fill defects after a lumpectomy, is also now commonplace. It may be possible soon to grow a whole breast from these fat 'stem cells'.

Lymphoedema is fortunately less common but if it occurs can be debilitating. Surgeons are beginning to offer lymph node transfer surgery and other techniques to try to treat this.

Advances in radiotherapy

There are two main advances in radiotherapy—establishing who can avoid it altogether, and if it is needed, can the side effects of it be minimized by targeting it better to the area of the breast where it is needed. It is already accepted that older women (over 70 years) with small good-outlook tumours may not need radiotherapy. However, trials are underway to try to define who younger than this may avoid it, perhaps by using molecular testing of the tumour.

Radiotherapy targeted to the tumour site only (partial breast radiotherapy) is increasingly accepted for women with lower risk tumours but radiotherapy still has the potential to cause long-term side effects. Ways of predicting and avoiding these are the topic of ongoing research.

New drug treatments for breast cancer

It is new drugs, and the biomarkers that go with them to predict in whom they will be effective, that is one of the most exciting new areas for research and advance.

Research into triple negative disease has led us to perhaps the most exciting advance in cancer in the last few years—our understanding of how the immune system interacts with cancers and how we can manipulate this. We are doing this in several ways. A group of drugs called immune checkpoint inhibitors (such as pembrolizumab and ipilimumab) have been discovered, which help the body's own immune system recognize the cancer cells as 'foreign' and attack them. These are effective in some cancers such as melanoma and are being trialled in breast cancer.

Other types of immune treatments being developed include cancer vaccines, CART-cell therapy (chimeric antigen receptor T cell) which may allow the T cells to better recognize cancer cells, and tumour-infiltrating lymphocytes (TIL) cell therapy (tumour-infiltrating lymphocyte) in which these TIL cells are removed from a cancer, treated to boost their ability to recognize cancer, and replaced into the patient to act as a 'silver bullet'. The role of micro-organisms living in our bodies, our microbiome, and how this interacts with our immune system, is perhaps the next frontier.

In the setting of hormone-receptor-positive breast cancer, new therapies that target the ER are still being developed. These include next-generation selective ER degraders that are more potent and orally administered. Other classes of targeted therapies are also being trialled in combination with endocrine therapies to circumvent endocrine resistance.

All cancer drugs have side effects. Important research is trying to minimize these side effects, and whether certain therapies can be de-escalated without inferior outcomes. For example, studies are evaluating if certain cardiac drugs, known as beta-blockers, can prevent the heart damage sometimes caused by the common breast cancer chemotherapy drugs, doxorubicin and epirubicin.

Better access to care

It is probably not a stretch to say that over the next decade we may not prevent breast cancer or cure all people who develop it—but for most, we will either be able to stop it spreading or for those who do have metastatic disease, we will be able to turn it into a chronic condition that rarely threatens life. Perhaps our greatest challenge will be to ensure all who develop breast cancer get easy access to excellent treatment no matter where they live. This will include how to translate the advances in care discovered in the developed world into better treatment for the many hundreds of thousands of patients—and numbers growing all the time—that develop breast cancer is less fortunate countries.

Further resources

American Cancer Society. *What's New in Breast Cancer Research?* Available at: https://www.cancer.org/cancer/breast-cancer/about/whats-new-in-breast-cancer-research.html

Breast Cancer Trials. Available at: https://www.breastcancertrials.org.au

Breastcancer.org. *Clinical Trials.* Available at: http://www.breastcancer.org/treatment/clinical_trials

Breastcancer.org. *What is Immunotherapy?* Available at: http://www.breastcancer.org/treatment/immunotherapy/what

NIH National Cancer Institute. *Clinical Trials Information for Patients and Caregivers.* Available at: https://www.cancer.gov/about-cancer/treatment/clinical-trials

Peter Mac. *iPrevent.* Available at: https://www.petermac.org\iprevent

Glossary

ADH See *Atypical ductal hyperplasia*

Adjuvant treatment Therapy after the initial treatment (i.e. extra treatment). In breast cancer, this usually means chemotherapy, radiotherapy, and/or hormonal therapy AFTER surgery.

Anaemia Deficiency in red blood cells/low blood count. This means less oxygen-carrying capacity in the blood and earlier fatigue. Anaemic patients can look pale.

Anastrazole Anti-oestrogen tablet used daily in postmenopausal women with oestrogen-sensitive breast cancer.

Angiogenic Forming new blood vessels. Cancers are angiogenic; they build new blood vessels to supply the growing tumour mass.

Antibodies Specialized proteins which recognize and attach to diseased cells helping the body's immune system attack them. While most antibodies are produced by our immune system, we can now create drugs which act as antibodies to help treat certain diseases including breast cancer. See *Immunotherapy*

Aromatase inhibitor (AI) Class of anti-oestrogen medications used in postmenopausal women with oestrogen-sensitive breast cancer. They block the hormone aromatase which is responsible for synthesizing oestrogen outside of the ovaries. Includes anastrazole, letrozole, and exemestane.

Atypia/Atypical Not normal. Abnormal.

Atypical ductal hyperplasia (ADH) Abnormal growth of breast milk duct cells which is a risk factor for, but does not constitute, breast cancer. Can be found nearby actual cancers and therefore surgical biopsy is usually recommended.

Atypical lobular hyperplasia (ALH) Like atypical ductal hyperplasia, but occurs in the milk-producing lobules in the breast tissue. ALH also indicates an increased risk of cancer but does not require surgery.

Axilla/axillary lymph nodes Axilla is the area between the chest and the arm, bounded front and back by muscles. Within this tissue are lymph nodes or glands, which filter fluid from the arm and breast on its way back into the blood. Cancer can spread along these lymphatic routes.

Axillary clearance Surgical removal of lymphatic tissue from the axilla.

Benign Not cancerous.

Bilateral Both left and right sides.

Biopsy Examination of a piece of tissue removed from the body in order to look for the presence and/or extent of disease. Biopsies can be taken via needle with the patient awake (see *Core biopsy* and *FNA*) or at surgery (see *Open surgical biopsy*).

Body mass index (BMI) A measure of whether someone is over or underweight derived from her height and weight.

Bone scan Type of scan assessing the bones for disease such as cancer spread.

BRCA (1 and/or 2) Breast cancer genes. These genes run in families and indicate a higher risk of breast, ovarian, and some other cancers in affected people.

Breast conserving therapy Surgery +/– radiotherapy in which the breast is preserved. An alternative to mastectomy for most breast cancers.

Breast reconstruction Surgical construction of a new breast after mastectomy, using various combinations of other body tissues and/or implants. Can be done at the time of mastectomy (immediate) or after treatment is concluded (delayed).

Cancer A group of diseases characterized by uncontrolled multiplication of abnormal cells from a given part of the body. Can be '*in situ*' or 'invasive'.

Carcinoma Cancer arising from the skin, or lining of internal organs. Breast carcinoma arises from the cells lining the milk-producing lobules and/or ducts.

CAR-T cell therapy CART-cell therapy (chimeric antigen receptor T cell) may allow the T cells to better recognize cancer cells

CDK 4/6 inhibitors A new class of anticancer drugs targeting cell division. Includes palbociclib, ribociclib, and abemaciclib.

Chemotherapy Also known as cytotoxic therapy. The treatment of disease via chemical substances (drugs) that kill cells.

Clinical trial Research comparing the effects of different treatments or of treatment versus no treatment in equivalent patient groups.

Complementary therapy Treatments which are used alongside conventional medical therapies to help manage symptoms and improve well-being.

Contrast Substance usually given by mouth or intravenously to enhance X-ray imaging techniques.

Core biopsy Needle biopsy in which a small piece of tissue can be removed from the patient. Usually done awake, under local anaesthetic, and can be guided by ultrasound or X-ray, CT, and even MRI as required.

CT scan Scan using multiple X-rays reconstructed on computer to create representative images of various cross sections (slices) of the body.

Cyst Thin-walled sacs containing fluid commonly found in the breast and other body tissues. In the breast, are usually insignificant and do not go on to become cancer.

DCIS (ductal carcinoma in situ) See *Ductal carcinoma in situ*

Deep inferior epigastric perforator (DIEP) flap Modern breast reconstruction technique, similar to a TRAM flap but sparing the abdominal muscle and thus using only abdominal skin and fat.

Disease-free survival The period for which a patient is free of cancer after treatment.

DNA Deoxyribonucleic acid. Molecules which code genetic information, present in essentially all our cells and necessary for them to grow, function, and reproduce.

Duct A tube or vessel. In the body, conveys fluid such as milk in the breast.

Ductal carcinoma in situ (DCIS) Breast cancer arising from duct cells, which is still confined within the duct system. A preinvasive breast cancer.

Embryo cryopreservation Removal and freezing of embryos (fertilized eggs) in order for later re-implantation into the uterus with the aim of pregnancy.

Endocrine therapy Treatment of hormone-sensitive breast cancer by depriving oestrogen and/or progesterone to the breast cancer cells.

Epigenetics The study of inheritable genetic changes where the underlying DNA is unchanged.

ER See *Oestrogen receptor*

Erythema Inflammation of the skin and other shallow tissues, showing up as redness and swelling. May be in response to injury, infection, or other irritation.

Estrogen See *Oestrogen*

Estrogen receptor (ER) See *Oestrogen receptor*

Excise/excision To surgically remove.

Familial breast cancer Breast cancer appearing in multiple family members—presumed secondary to a transmitted ('passed along') breast cancer gene.

Fibroadenoma Benign breast tumour made up of glandular and fibrous tissue. Typically occurs in younger women and is not a risk factor for breast cancer.

Fine needle aspiration (FNA) Technique to sample cells and/or fluid from a cyst, solid mass, or lymph node via a thin needle. Usually done with the patient awake, with or without ultrasound guidance.

Genes Hereditary material that provides instructions for the body on how to build all cells and tissues. Can carry various characteristics through families.

Gene mutations Abnormalities in a gene, which may be passed on from parent to offspring or may be occur spontaneously. Can lead to cells and tissues growing or functioning abnormally, manifesting as cancer or other disease.

Gonadotrophin-releasing hormone (GnRH) analogues Drugs which trick the pituitary gland into reducing production of luteinizing hormone (LH), which is required by the ovaries to drive oestrogen production. This puts the ovaries to 'sleep', creating a reversible menopause. Includes goserelin and tryptorelin.

Grade A way of classifying cancers according to their appearance. Low-grade cancers have a lower risk of recurrence as opposed to high-grade cancers. Breast cancers are typically graded from 1 (low) to 3 (high).

Her2 receptor Also known as 'cErbB-2'. Stands for human epidermal growth factor receptor and is overactive on ~20% of breast cancers. The target of anti-Her2 'immunotherapy' drugs like Herceptin.

Herceptin Also known as trastuzumab. A newer type of treatment which is not chemotherapy, but which works well with chemotherapy against Her2-positive breast cancer. See *Immunotherapy*

Histology Microscopic analysis of tissues.

Hookwire localization Technique of placing a wire into the breast under X-ray or ultrasound guidance to help the surgeon find lesions he or she otherwise can't feel to then remove.

Hormonal therapy See *Endocrine therapy*

Hormone receptor A molecule in the breast cancer cell that is 'switched on' by the attachment of oestrogen or progesterone and may facilitate further growth/multiplication.

Hormone replacement therapy (HRT) Oestrogen and/or progesterone given to reduce the effects of menopause.

Hysterectomy Surgical removal of the uterus (womb).

IDC See *Invasive ductal carcinoma*

ILC See *Invasive lobular carcinoma*

Immune checkpoint inhibitors These are drugs (such as pembrolizumab and ipilimumab) which help the body's own immune system recognize the cancer cells as 'foreign' and attack them.

Immunotherapy Treatments which stimulate the body's very powerful immune system to destroy cancer cells which otherwise may be 'hiding'. Includes drugs which act as antibodies to the Her2 receptor. See *Herceptin*, *Perjeta*, and *Immune checkpoint inhibitors*

Impalpable Undetectable by touch alone.

Imprint cytology A laboratory technique for rapid microscopic assessment of surgical and other tissue specimens.

Inflammatory breast cancer A type of locally advanced breast cancer that presents with a red, warm, and swollen breast often with peau d'orange.

In situ In its original place. With regard to cancer, this indicates preinvasive change—see *Ductal carcinoma in situ (DCIS)*

Internal mammary nodes Lymph nodes or glands sitting behind the breastbone. Tissue fluid from the breast drains primarily to axillary lymph nodes but can also drain centrally to these nodes

Invasive Spreading beyond usual boundaries. With breast cancer, this can refer to direct spread into surrounding tissues or more distant spread via lymphatic and/or blood vessels.

Invasive ductal carcinoma (IDC) Most common type of breast cancer, originating in the milk ducts and making up about 75% of all breast cancer. May also be described as 'not otherwise specified (NOS)' or 'no special type (NST)', as it is a very typical looking cancer under the microscope.

Invasive lobular carcinoma (ILC) Second most common type of breast cancer, originating in the milk-producing part of the breast (lobule) and making up about 15% of all breast cancer.

In vitro fertilization (IVF) Production of an embryo—that is, fertilization of an egg by sperm—taking place outside the body (i.e. in a test tube).

Latissimus dorsi (LD) flap Breast reconstruction technique utilizing muscle, fat, and skin from the back, often in conjunction with an implant for adequate bulk.

LCIS See *Lobular carcinoma in situ*

Lipomodelling Where fat is sucked out of the tummy or thigh and injected over a reconstruction or to fill defects after a lumpectomy. Also known as lipofilling or fat grafting.

Lobular carcinoma in situ (LCIS) Abnormal but non-cancerous growth of cells lining the breast lobule (milk-producing unit). Indicates a higher risk of future breast cancer.

Lobule Part of an organ. The breast is made up of milk-producing units known as lobules.

Locally advanced breast cancer (LABC) Cancers which have any combination of the following: >5 cm, growing into skin, muscle, or bone, causing other skin change such as erythema or peau d'orange, and/or spread to multiple lymph nodes.

Lumpectomy Surgical excision of a breast lump or other lesion, which may be for diagnostic purposes or to alleviate symptoms. The breast is otherwise conserved. (Lumpectomy may be used in the context of breast-preserving cancer excision, although this should more properly be referred to as wide local excision.)

LVI See *Lymphovascular invasion*

Lymph Body tissue fluid, bathing the cells at all times.

Lymph nodes/glands Glands within the lymphatic system which act as filtering or cleansing stations for lymph as it is ferried through the lymphatic vessels from the body's tissues back into the bloodstream.

Lymphoedema Chronic swelling of a body part due to inadequate removal of lymph by the lymphatic system. In breast cancer, lymphoedema most commonly affects the arm after surgery or radiotherapy to the axillary lymph glands.

Lymphovascular invasion Spread of cancer cells into blood and/or lymphatic vessels.

Magnetic resonance imaging (MRI) Scan using a magnetic field rather than X-rays to produce internal pictures of the body. Increasingly used in screening for breast cancer in high-risk women, as well as assessing more complicated breast cancers preoperatively.

Malignant Cancerous. See *Cancer*

Mammogram Breast X-ray.

Mammogram tomosynthesis Newer type of mammogram creating a 3D rather than 2D picture of the breast to provide greater chance of detecting breast cancer.

Margin The amount of normal tissue around the diseased area in a surgically removed lesion.

Mastalgia Breast pain.

Mastectomy Surgical removal of all breast tissue on one side.

Medical oncologist Specialist who uses chemotherapy and other medications in the treatment of cancer.

Menarche The onset of menstruation—a female's first 'period'.

Menopause The cessation of menstrual periods—typically at around 50 years of age.

Metastasis/metastases/metastatic Cancerous growths distant from the initial cancer.

Microarray technology A pathology technique which aims to make a 'fingerprint' of the molecular changes in a tissue.

Microcalcifications The deposition of calcium into tissues. In the breast, this can be a marker of cancerous change and shows up as white dots on mammogram.

MRI See *Magnetic resonance imaging*

Multidisciplinary (meeting)/MDM The involvement of multiple medical specialists from different but complimentary areas, along with para-medical staff to create and facilitate the best possible treatment plan for a patient with complex disease such as cancer.

Nausea Feeling of sickness with inclination to vomit.

Neoadjuvant treatment Treatment such as chemotherapy, radiotherapy, or hormonal therapy given prior to surgery in an attempt to make the latter more successful.

Neoplasm Abnormal growth of a tissue within the body. Can be malignant or benign.

Nodal status Whether cancer has spread to nearby lymph nodes. In breast cancer, this usually refers to the status of the axillary nodes.

Oestrogen Hormone, which promotes and maintains female characteristics.

Oestrogen receptor (ER) A molecule in the breast cancer cell that is 'switched on' by the attachment of oestrogen and may facilitate further growth/multiplication.

Oncologist Doctor specializing in cancer treatment. There are three main types: medical, radiation, and surgical oncologist.

Oophorectomy Surgical removal of the ovaries to reduce oestrogen levels in bringing forward menopause and/or to reduce the risk of ovarian cancer.

Open surgical biopsy Biopsy performed via a cut in the operating theatre. Surgical biopsy may be excisional (removing the entire lesion of interest) or incisional (removing a piece of a larger area of concern).

Osteoporosis A weakening of the bones that occurs with age and may be worsened by factors such as hormonal changes, lack of exercise, and dietary imbalance.

Ovarian ablation Stopping of ovarian function either by removal at surgery or by radiotherapy. Irreversible.

Ovarian suppression Temporary cessation of ovarian function via administration of drugs such as the gonadotrophin-releasing hormone (GnRH) analogues.

Palliative care Treatment aimed at alleviating pain and other problems associated with an advanced and terminal disease state.

Palpable Detectable by touch.

Papilloma/papillary lesion In the breast, these are growths, usually benign, but occasionally cancerous. Surgical excision is usually recommended due to the small possibility of cancer.

PARP inhibitors An experimental therapy, which may be effective in treating breast cancers in *BRCA* gene carriers and potentially other patients also. 'PARP' means poly (ADP ribose) polymerase and is involved in the repair of certain cells after damage.

Partial breast irradiation An experimental radiotherapy technique that aims to treat only the part of the breast affected by cancer.

Pathology/pathologist The study of disease. 'Pathology' can specifically refer to the type of disease within a given individual: 'her pathology shows … '. A doctor specializing in pathology is a pathologist.

Peau d'orange French for the 'skin of an orange'. When the breast develops this swollen and discoloured appearance, it can be a sign of underlying cancer.

Perjeta Also known as pertuzumab. Like *Herceptin*, an immunotherapy drug targeting the Her2 receptor in Her2 positive breast cancer.

Pertuzumab See *Perjeta*

PET scan Full body scan looking for areas of high metabolism (measured by glucose consumption). Tumours are often revealed as they tend to be metabolically very active.

PR See *Progesterone receptor*

Preinvasive Cells, which while similar in appearance to invasive cancer cells, have not yet gained the ability to invade beyond their usual surrounds. See *Ductal carcinoma in situ (DCIS)* and *In situ*

Progesterone Hormone, which stimulates and regulates various female functions including menstruation and pregnancy.

Progesterone receptor (PR) A molecule in the breast cancer cell that is 'switched on' by the attachment of progesterone and may facilitate further growth/multiplication.

Prognosis The likely outcome of a disease in an individual, based on outcomes of similar patients.

Prophylactic mastectomy Mastectomy performed when cancer is not present but to reduce the risk of it occurring by removing breast tissue pre-emptively.

Prothesis Artificial body part such as an arm, leg or in the case of breast cancer, an artificial breast worn in the bra after mastectomy.

Radial scar Benign breast lesion which can mimic breast cancer. Surgical excision is usually recommended.

Radiation oncologist Specialist who uses radiotherapy in the treatment of cancer.

Radical or modified radical mastectomy Operations for breast cancer, involving removal of the breast as well as lymph glands from the axilla, and in the radical option, some chest muscles.

Radiology/Radiologist The study of body imaging including with X-ray and ultrasound. A doctor specializing in radiology is a radiologist.

Radiotherapy Treatment of disease using radiation.

Receptor A part of a cell which responds to a specific stimulus, creating secondary effects in the cell.

Recurrent cancer Relapse of cancer after a patient has been disease free for a period.

Re-excision Surgical removal of further tissue when initial tissue fails to remove a cancerous area with clear margin.

Relapse See *Recurrent cancer*

Remission Reduction in the severity of disease. Can be partial or complete and temporary or permanent.

Risk factor Something which increases the likelihood of developing a particular disease or condition.

Screening A medical test or other strategy recommended to a selected population to detect disease where there are no other symptoms.

Sentinel lymph node biopsy (SNB) Surgical removal of the first lymph gland/s the breast drains to in order to determine whether cancer has spread there, which may necessitate removal of further glands.

Seroma Collection of inflammatory fluid under the skin after surgery, which may require needle drainage intermittently.

Simple mastectomy Mastectomy without removal of any axillary lymph glands.

Skin sparing or subcutaneous mastectomy Mastectomy with preservation of overlying skin +/- nipple and areola, for use in immediate breast reconstruction.

Sporadic Happening without any pattern. Occurring unpredictably.

Staging Determination of the extent of cancer in the body.

Supraclavicular nodes Lymph glands in the area above the collarbone.

Surgical biopsy See *Open surgical biopsy*

Survivorship The long-term issues for women following a diagnosis of cancer and the treatment for it.

Systemic treatment Treatments such as chemotherapy and hormonal therapy which are aimed at disease anywhere in the body, as opposed to surgery and radiotherapy which target specific areas where the disease load is greatest.

Tamoxifen (TAM) Anti-oestrogen medication given daily, used in premenopausal women with hormone-sensitive breast cancers. It may also have a role in cancer prevention in some women.

Tissue expander Temporary expandable implant used in breast reconstruction surgery to gradually stretch up the tissues for the final implant, placed at a second operation.

Tissue flap Tissue taken from elsewhere in the body, for use in various functions at the disease site; for example, breast reconstruction after mastectomy. See *Latissimus dorsi (LD)* and *Transverse rectus abdominis muscle (TRAM)* flap reconstruction

Transverse rectus abdominis muscle (TRAM) flap Breast reconstruction technique utilizing muscle, fat, and skin from the abdomen.

Trastuzumab See *Herceptin*

Triple receptor negative breast cancer Breast cancer which is ER-, PR-, and Her2-receptor negative.

Triple test Clinical (verbal and physical), radiological (mammogram, ultrasound, and so on) and biopsy assessment of concerning breast lesions, which is recommended to minimize the chance of missing cancer.

Tumour See *Neoplasm*

Ultrasound Method of radiologically assessing lesions within the body by the use of ultrasonic waves.

Wide local excision Surgical excision of a cancer, as well as a margin of normal tissue around it. In breast cancer surgery, wide local excision is an alternate to mastectomy for smaller cancers.

Index

Notes *vs.* indicates a comparison
Tables and figures are indicated by an italic *t* or *f* following the page number.